India Knight's Beauty Edit

India Knight is the author of five novels: *Darling, Mutton, Comfort and Joy, Don't You Want Me?* and *My Life on a Plate*. She is a columnist for the *Sunday Times*, and she lives in Suffolk.

India Knight's Beauty Edit

What Works When You're Older

INDIA KNIGHT

FIG TREE
an imprint of
PENGUIN BOOKS

FIG TREE

UK | USA | Canada | Ireland | Australia
India | New Zealand | South Africa

Fig Tree is part of the Penguin Random House group of companies
whose addresses can be found at global.penguinrandomhouse.com

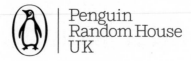

First published 2023
001

Set in 13.5/16pt Garamond MT Std
Typeset by Jouve (UK), Milton Keynes
Printed and bound in Great Britain by Clays Ltd, Elcograf S.p.A.

The authorized representative in the EEA is Penguin Random House Ireland,
Morrison Chambers, 32 Nassau Street, Dublin D02 YH68

A CIP catalogue record for this book is available from the British Library

ISBN: 978–0–241–67255–6

www.greenpenguin.co.uk

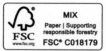

Penguin Random House is committed to a
sustainable future for our business, our readers
and our planet. This book is made from Forest
Stewardship Council® certified paper.

Contents

CONTENTS

PART 3

The Extras Edit

Introduction

So here we are, older, having lived a whole lot of life, having learned a whole lot of valuable stuff the hard way, and still in a position to make good use of our findings. We know what's what. We know what to care and not care about. We're wise, or at least wiser. We're strong as bears. We're amazing. I love us.

But I don't love that we're also often newly insecure about the way ageing manifests in our faces, and what we should do about it. Anything? Nothing? Denial? Acceptance? It's as if the trusty autopilot we relied on for decades has gone rogue: what looked great for years suddenly looks . . . less great. Now what?

Sometimes it feels like the choice is starkly binary. Option A is setting off on the path that ultimately leads to looking like current-era Madonna – a defiant, poignant clinging to youth via cosmetic procedures, some of which are playfully called 'tweakments' as if they were cute, fun little nothings. Option B is going for the full pottery-teacher look, in a smock and a bare face and maybe some 'jazzy' earrings. (No offence to pottery teachers – this, minus the jazzier aspects, is pretty much my daily look, especially when I'm at my pottery classes.)

What we all want is the sane, considered middle way:

the best version of us at the age we are. It sounds simple. It is not simple. We used to know what to buy, how to do our makeup, and what to put on our skin, but what was once second nature – open the makeup bag and this goes here, and that goes there, and I like putting this on like that, done, let's go – is now more challenging. I wore flicky black liquid eyeliner most days from the age of fifteen to when I was about fifty, to the point where I could practically put it on in the dark, until one day it just didn't work any more. It didn't look right. I hadn't changed, and my love of flicky black liquid eyeliner hadn't changed. But my eyes had. The liner brush now had to travel across significantly more rugged terrain. Those new creases made it harder to apply neatly, and because – yay – my eyelids are more hooded than they used to be, the eyeliner wasn't properly visible when I had my eyes open.*

So what? you may ask. Well, so I had stopped looking like myself to my own eyes, and that is a very discombobulating thing. An eroded sense of self does not make for being comfortable in one's skin, and is therefore deleterious to women's happiness. It matters. I mourned the me who had always worn liner. The linerless me had eyes that looked unmoored, floating about my face, undefined and naked-looking. It made me feel sad.

You'll have your own version of my eyeliner: the lipstick that always used to look great, until it didn't because

* There is a solution to this problem. It is on page 259.

your lips had thinned. The reliable foundation that now makes your skin look kind of dead. The eyeshadow that once glided on but now migrates to creases and sits there stubbornly. The once-reliable concealer that's started saying, 'Hi! Let me just really emphasize your pores.'

When I talk to friends of my age and older about beauty later in life, pretty much everyone mentions having once had a look, *their* look, that they could pull out of the bag no matter what, and how that look no longer quite works for them, and the feelings of sorrow and loss it engenders. What makes it worse is that they have no idea of what they should replace the lost look with. 'Do I just wear beige everything now?' one friend asked. 'Or grey? Because it's not really me. The me in my head is wearing metallic eyeshadow and wispy lashes, but obviously I can't do that either because I'd look tragic. Wouldn't I? I literally don't have a clue. Also, am I too old for contour? What *is* contour?'

The other issue that always comes up is choice. As in there's too much of it. You just want a mascara, but there are three thousand on offer. It makes you exhausted just thinking about it. How are you supposed to choose, not just with mascaras but more generally? There are hundreds of thousands, millions, of beauty products out there. Are they even any cop at this stage of life, or do they, like the department-store Santa in *Elf*, sit on a throne of lies? It gets particularly confusing with skincare, when the trend is for minimalist labelling that often tells you only the chemical name of the contents, like 'succinic acid treatment' or 'tranexamid acid serum'. You what?

Also in the mix: we're no longer sure about what we're 'supposed' to look like. Our fifty or sixty or seventy isn't our mothers' fifty or sixty or seventy, which is cheering, and the sense that older women should quietly put themselves out to pasture is eroding (quite slowly, it must be said). There's something else at play, too. My generation and the ones before it, stretching back to the mists of time, were brought up to be found pleasing by men, to welcome or at least not mind the male gaze, to strive never to look anything other than our most desirable best. This was part and parcel of our sense of self.

We learned by societal osmosis that we had some sort of duty to be as aesthetically pleasing as was humanly possible, to primp and depilate and paint until we were 'presentable', or, more bluntly, fanciable: attractive to strangers. In my first novel, written in 1999, the narrator's mother tells her that she has 'let herself go' following marriage and having children. It was kind of a joke, and also kind of not. Twenty-five years on, I work from home, mostly in no makeup, jogging bottoms and old sweaters, and it took me an embarrassingly long time to stop making jokes about how unglamorous and rustic I looked when anyone dropped in. I know that looking glamorous isn't my job. But that stuff, hardwired from childhood, lingers stubbornly. It's a primal fear: do I look unsexy? Oh, my God, do I look *old*?

I notice by contrast that many younger women know exactly what they think of the male gaze. They think it can go and shove itself. They don't derive a misplaced sense of approval, let alone much of their identity, from being found pleasing by total strangers: they couldn't care less about being deemed attractive by random men they don't know and have no interest in knowing. Being ogled is an aggression rather than mildly flattering. And so it follows that you can tell people's age, even if they're coy about it, by their attitude to beauty and, always, diet (hence the eighty-five-year-old who won't have cake because it'll make her 'fat'). It's an older person's mindset: the duty to please, even if it means you're hungry.

I hate the idea of trying desperately to look less old to please other people. There is nothing wrong with looking older, just as there is nothing wrong with eating the cake. (Eat the sodding cake! Embrace pleasure! Time is marching on!) The book you're holding isn't trying to turn back time or make anyone look improbable or weird. Neither is it saying that women 'should' do anything at all, although in my view we *should* all have a really great skincare routine, regardless of whether we do or don't wear makeup. This book's purpose is to make older women feel and look better in relation to things that might disconcert them about their appearance, and to identify the things that they – we – can actually do something about.

I have tried to make my advice relevant and useful for women of all ethnic (I hate that word but it's the right

one here) backgrounds, which is to say for all skin colours. I am of mixed Pakistani and Belgian heritage. I
wasn't able to buy foundation that matched my skin
colour until I was in my twenties. Even then it was
expensive, custom-blended and not available outside big
cities. The effect was to make me feel, throughout my
teens and early twenties, as if the skin colour I was proud
of was some sort of deeply bizarre anomaly. That's not
a good feeling for any young woman to have.

It would be another ten years before big commercial
brands started offering products in a broader range of
shades and another twenty before those shades felt like
anything more than a box-ticking exercise. Today, more
than thirty years later, Black women whose skin is very
dark still routinely find that even brands that trumpet
their inclusivity aren't always able to cater to their needs.
Not feeling seen is soul-destroying. Do any cosmetics
brands really want to be saying, 'We're for everybody
except you,' in the twenty-first century?*

I am also massively against the idea that not using
makeup or cosmetics is somehow a dereliction of duty.
It can be a fantastic liberation, too, especially if you are
of the generations I described above, so used to the
relentless gaze of the patriarchy and so hardwired to be

---

* Having said all of that – and, man, I could say a lot more – I must point
out that my knowledge is necessarily subjective. I do not have East Asian
heritage, and I am not Black. Any mistakes or omissions in this book are
mine.

found 'pleasing' by it at all times that your whole sense of self depends on it. All of that is a given. But you can still dislike your ageing neck and wonder if there's any meaningful action you can take, and you can still occasionally fancy wearing a fantastic lipstick just for the heck of it. You know? The world is heavy. Gloom is everywhere. Beauty products are light. Everybody needs a little glam and frivolity every now and then, a little luxurious, treat-feeling, unapologetic fun to take them away from the bleakness of the endlessly grim news cycle, or from whatever other challenges are going on in their life (the list often starts with the double whammy of ailing parents and tricky teenagers). You could even call it self-care.

Here's how I think about it: for older women, makeup used to be the equivalent of a sweetshop, stuffed full of appetizing and recognizable favourites. But now the friendly sweetshop has closed and been replaced with a gigantic megamall filled with hundreds of thousands of baffling options, all promising the moon, all leaving you giddy and exhausted with choice. So the temptation is to stick with what you know – to sit there sadly with your dusty stash – or not to bother any more because you're too old, there's nothing to be done and it's all too confusing.

That would be a mistake. New formulations and technological advances have reinvented both makeup and skincare and made both dramatically more effective. What this book seeks to do is to open the megamall

7

especially for you, take you by the hand and lead you straight to the good stuff that works. There are new things, a few old things, and alternatives to all the products you liked before they stopped working/sat in your lines/emphasized your sun damage. With beauty as with so much else, knowledge is power. Here's all of mine.

Note 1. Cosmetics have an annoying habit of getting discontinued or reformulated. My recommendations should be good for at least a few years after publication. I have also explained *why* things work, so I hope that even if something were discontinued, you would feel confident enough to find a replacement.

Note 2. There are hundreds of thousands of beauty products in the world and obviously it would be impossible for one person, or even a hundred people, to test every single one. If your favourites don't appear in the following pages, it isn't necessarily because I don't rate them. My criterion for inclusion was really simple: products tested on myself that are so effective I would (and do) buy them with my own money when the press samples run out.

PART 1
Skincare

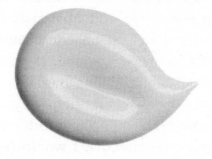

Skincare is everything. Good skin is what makes you look in good nick. Seriously. Be French about it: this is where you should spend your money. There's a big caveat, though: don't spend too much of it by making the (understandable) mistake of thinking that the more you cough up the better the product is. This is not the case, or at least it's only sometimes the case. By way of illustration, I have a friend who is currently launching a skincare line. It has been put together by the most esteemed and knowledgeable chemists and skincare experts imaginable. There's a particularly effective face cream, packed full of absolutely top-notch ingredients.

Here's the thing: it's cheap to make, as in the cream itself is cheap. What's expensive is the packaging. Brands recoup this expense and more via their (wild) mark-ups. So don't be seduced by a massive price tag, thinking, 'It must be worth it. They wouldn't dare otherwise.' They would and they do. What you are usually paying for is a beautiful, desirable packaging aesthetic – great if you can afford it, not a problem in terms of actually caring for your skin if you can't. Equally, don't be seduced by waiting lists, which are normally figments of the marketing team's imagination but which obviously become self-fulfilling when enough people bite. If you're rich, it's of course lovely to have a luxurious, expensively scented face cream in a weighty glass jar – but you're usually paying more for the glass jar than for the cream. (At the time of writing, the price of glass has gone off the charts. You never really think about the price of glass, do you, apart from if you're buying windows? But it's a thing. It fluctuates a lot, recently by 50 per cent at a time.)

The pricing situation applies across the board. Unless you are very concerned about how things look on your bathroom shelf, you don't need to pay top whack. Having said that, some products come in dark or amber glass jars because the contents thrive in the absence of light and because glass stays cool, like a fridge, rather than like a sweaty plastic tube in a warm or hot bathroom. And some products are expensive, despite their inexpensive packaging, because they can be, because they're really good. But they are few and far between.

Here's a rule I abide by: if in doubt, go for a French pharmacy brand. It's never going to be a bad choice. My absolute favourite is Bioderma – it's incredibly reliable across the board – closely followed by La Roche-Posay. Both have specific ranges addressing specific concerns.

Please remember, though, that unless we're talking about very powerful ingredients, skincare doesn't effect transformations overnight. It takes time. You have to stick with it. When I am testing a product for my column, I use it for at least four weeks before writing it up.

But let's start at the beginning, with cleansing.

PART 1
Skincare

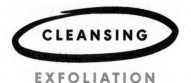
CLEANSING

EXFOLIATION

SERUMS

MOISTURIZERS

OILY OR SPOT-PRONE SKIN

SUN DAMAGE AND SUN SPOTS

TWEAKMENTS

AT-HOME TREATMENTS

EYES

NECKS

Apparently the actress Cameron Diaz has stopped washing her face. This isn't some weird rumour: she said so herself on a BBC podcast. 'I literally do nothing. I, like, never wash my face . . . Twice a month, if I'm lucky, I'll be like, "Oh, I better put this on. One time works, right?"' I've tried to decide if she was exaggerating for comic effect, but I don't think so – and, anyway, outing yourself as terminally grubby is not especially comedic: 'Yeah, I never brush my teeth, lol.' On the other hand, Diaz has been loudly and laudably outspoken in the past about the ludicrous expectations the film industry has about how women should look. I applaud her for this – but, Jeez, Cam, wash your face! Do it for yourself! Not washing your face is gross. (Conversely, not washing your hair can be quite effective.)

Or it could be that it was a way of saying, 'All this hair and makeup that is supposedly central to what makes a woman – it's literally got nothing to do with it'? But then you'd say, 'I hate makeup,' not 'I never wash my face.'

'I never wash my face' is to me about two degrees away from some incel type saying, 'I find the genitals are self-cleaning.' It's really not at all good at any level. Still, I resent the amount of time I have spent wondering about Diaz's face and the accruing sebum thereon. Onwards to cleansers.

Regardless of skin type, I very strongly favour balms and oils, to the exclusion of anything else, for the simple reasons that (a) they get everything off, (b) they're gentle, glide and never drag, and (c) they never dry your skin out. This is really important always, but especially in middle age and beyond, when retaining moisture is a non-negotiable necessity and where 'squeaky-clean', as in almost audibly stripped, is the enemy. Your skin is basically a camel in the Sahara, permanently looking for oases. Any cleanser that makes your face feel even the slightest bit tight, so that it isn't entirely comfortable until you apply moisturizer, is a bad cleanser or – let's be generous – simply not the cleanser for you.

I am a balm devotee. I love them. I love using them, I love what they do, I love the way they make your skin feel, and I love how clean they get it without it ever feeling tight (Elemis and Amanda Lacey for preference, for me, but there are lots of others at every price).

Sometimes people worry that their skin won't get on with an oily cleanser (a balm is merely a solidified oily concoction) because it's congested or prone to breakouts, or it's combination, with an oily T-zone, or oily *tout court*. I agree with the idea that oil upon oil is a weird and potentially disastrous concept, but that's not how it plays out. Have faith. Also, be aware that sometimes the skin overproduces grease or sebum because it's so parched and is frantically trying to lubricate itself.

If you have any teenagers about your person whose skin is driving them to despair, it is worth reminding them of this. Nothing harsh, ever. That applies in triplicate to older women – not because of an excess of hormones, in our case, but because of the opposite. Everything we do is about keeping moisture in and adding more on top for good measure. Think of your skin as a lovely old – let's say 'vintage': it sounds nicer – handbag. You don't leave it to dry out all by itself. You lovingly nourish it with – well, with a product called dubbin, which is what soldiers use on their boots and which is the best thing for restoring shine and flex to tired leather. But you get the idea: you lubricate handbags, and you lubricate skin, and suppleness returns and is maintained.

I use cleansers at night with either a pristinely clean muslin cloth or, for preference, an old-fashioned pristinely clean flannel. In the morning, I wipe my face with the same muslin/flannel soaked in hot water – no product. (Afterwards the flannel goes in the wash. I buy them in bulk to avoid putting the washing machine on too often.) Obviously this doubles the life of your cleanser, but that's not why I do it. I do it because I am wary of overloading skin with stuff it doesn't need. I really passionately believe that skin needs to breathe, just as it is, with nothing else on it. If you really have to deep-wash your face in the morning because you're just back from the gym or have for some reason woken up really grubby, use a very small amount of something at the cheaper end of the scale, like CeraVe.

Here's how I judge a new cleanser. It has to be nice to use, obviously; it has to get every last scrap of dirt and makeup off; it has to leave my skin feeling pleasantly plump and hydrated; but most of all I have to wake up and notice a pleasing and visible improvement. This improvement should be evident not just the next morning – because that's more about your skin going, 'Ooh, newness! Let's show willing,' than about tangible long-term benefits – but also 'going forward', to use a loathsome phrase.

THE EDIT: SEVEN
BRILLIANT CLEANSERS

- **Emma Lewisham Illuminating Oil Cleanser (around £55)**. A recent discovery, and one I hadn't expected to fall in love with. I was basically having a quick drink to be polite and hoping to be home in time for *The Archers*. But in the manner of these things, it didn't turn out that way. This did everything I ask for in a cleanser in absolute spades. The improvement the next morning was noticeable, the improvement over the next week really quite startling. It's not cheap, but it's a very, very good product indeed.
- **Elemis Pro-Collagen Cleansing Balm (around £48)**. Beloved by me for well over a decade: whatever else I'm testing, I come back

to this like a homing pigeon. Leaves skin perfectly clean, comfortable and soothed. Also comes in a fragrance-free Naked version. You need only a tiny pea-sized amount.

- **The Body Shop Camomile Sumptuous Makeup Cleaning Butter (around £6)**. Lovely on the skin, including sensitive, this is particularly effective if you wear a lot of makeup. The Body Shop, which had fallen out of fashion, has had a major revamp and is now always worth looking at for well-priced, effective skincare that punches well above its price tag.
- In the high street, see also **Lush Ultrabland (around £20)**, which is excellent on drier skins. Like the Body Shop cleanser above, this does as good a job at removing every last scrap of makeup as products three times the price.
- **Trinny London Be Your Best Balm (around £32)** contains lots of fruit enzymes to eat away dead cells.
- **DHC Deep Cleansing Oil (around £27)**. This, from a Japanese brand, has been around for ever, outlived many imitators, and remains fantastic. Olive-oil based.
- **CeraVe cleansers** are excellent. I particularly like the **Foaming Oil Cleanser** with hyaluronic acid **(around £14)**.

REMOVING EYE MAKEUP

All of the above cleansers, being oily, will remove ordinary amounts of eye makeup effectively. If you've really piled it on, I would remove the worst of it with a cotton pad or six soaked in micellar water. This is water that contains a tiny amount of a cleansing agent – detergent – that forms large micelles (clusters of molecules). The large micelles do a better job than middling micelles, small micelles or tiny micelles. Micellar water is gentle and doesn't sting, is good on both sensitive and spot-prone skin, and is inexpensive. My favourite, because contrary to popular belief they are not all the same (since the detergent component varies), is **Sensibio H2O by Bioderma (around £20)**. If you prefer a dedicated eye makeup remover, I love **Gatineau Floracil Gentle Eye Makeup Remover (around £35 for a giant bottle)**, which is cooling enough to feel slightly like a compress, is not remotely oily and gets every last scrap off. It's fantastic on waterproof mascara but, crucially, gentle enough to use on eyelash extensions (and see page 240 for more about those). Gatineau actually discontinued this remover, but there was such a massive outcry that they reinstated it, and in jumbo bottles. A little goes a long way as it's so effective, which in my view is a better combination than the false economy of using something cheap in vast quantities.

In the end, you know your own skin best. As long as you don't do a Cameron Diaz and decide it doesn't need washing at all, use what you feel works for you. If you're happy using soap, Johnson's Baby Oil (I know, but a friend does this and has amazing skin, to my permanent astonishment), a cream cleanser that you wipe off with cotton wool, or that trusty old stalwart, cold cream – which still has its fans* – then you carry right on. One of the tyrannies of the beauty industry is that it always encourages you to think that something significantly better than what you're using exists – even if you only bought your new cleanser, or whatever, last week. It's this sort of thing that keeps women in a state of low-level anxiety about getting it 'wrong'.

* It's effectively a water-and-fat emulsion, and therefore theoretically not so different from many more modern cleansers. Avoid on oilier skins.

PART 1
Skincare

Acids, peels and the rest

First things first: nothing has ever exfoliated my skin better than gentle daily scrubbing with a flannel. I'd go as far as saying that doing this changed my skin, in that it categorically sorted out a mildly congested T-zone, which never came back. I was familiar with the idea of cleaning your face with a muslin, thanks to Eve Lom the person, who popularized the method in the mid-1980s. But I thought you had to be very reverent and pat politely rather than really get in there, and I couldn't understand why this transformative method of cleansing transformed everyone's skin except mine. So in case this is you: if you use a muslin or a flannel, really insist on areas like the sides of the nose, the chin, the bit between your eyebrows, or anywhere else that feels like it could be clearer and smoother. You want to apply enough pressure to your flannel to feel it – go round in little circles where possible – but obviously not so much that your face is all red. As I mentioned in the previous chapter, use a fresh flannel daily. Doing this and drinking more water are the two best things I've done for my skin. It is very, very boring to drone on about drinking more water, so I won't, but – it makes a huge difference.

Having said all that, it is a fact that pretty much all skin benefits from a more thorough exfoliation every now and then. Think of heels, knees or elbows, or anywhere else where stubbornly dry skin congregates: softening these areas isn't simply a question of rubbing in the richest cream you can find, because you'd be rubbing it on dead skin that's formed an impenetrable layer and nothing much would happen. A much less dramatic (thank goodness) version of this takes place on the face too. Skin is constantly shedding and the dead cells quite like sitting around long after they should have made an exit, like the drunk person who won't leave even though you're in your pyjamas and are turning out all the lights. You need to get it off, not least so that any products you use can actually get to work.

In my young-personhood, exfoliation meant scratching away at your face with scrubs containing grit in the form of things like apricot kernels. These still exist, incredibly. The other day my friend A, who is out and about in the world and does not live under a rock, asked me to recommend her a gritty exfoliant. I said, 'What do you mean, a gritty exfoliant? Are we fourteen? Do you want to borrow my Anne French cleanser while you're at it?' (Nostalgic pause as we light a memory-candle for dear Anne French cleanser, which actually needs no candle as it still exists.)

'What's wrong with gritty exfoliants?' said A, snippily. 'I just wondered if you could point me to a good one.'

So then it occurred to me that perhaps some people still exfoliate in the twentieth-century manner, which would be harmless if it didn't mean (a) scratching your face half to death – like scouring delicate china with some sort of janitorial XXL industrial scrubber – and (b) having at some point contributed to the microbead horror. It's particularly silly because neither of these things is necessary. Gritty exfoliants work by being gritty, as when the Fairy Liquid isn't enough and you need one of the green scouring pads.

What you want instead is a liquid exfoliant – a toner, a gel, a face wash or a serum – which does the job far more effectively and doesn't literally scratch the surface of your skin. They are a gazillion trillion times more effective. They can make you look like you've had a light version of a peel, i.e. like you have new skin. It is as though you'd been scrubbing away at your grotty old pan with burned-on bits for years, crying, and somebody just comes along in the night and leaves you a brand-new Le Creuset.

This is where we get into the realm of acids, which confuse a lot of people. The first thing to know is that using any of these products makes your skin more vulnerable to sun damage, so always, always wear sunscreen while you're using them or you'll get brown spots and worse. Using acids will inevitably reveal new skin, hurrah, but that new skin, being new, will be delicate and vulnerable. I never use acids in the summer, when I'm outside in the sun for much of the day. This is probably overly paranoid, but better safe than sorry. You only get one face. For the same reason, use your exfoliating products at night.

Here's a quick explainer.

- **Alpha hydroxy acids, or AHAs, get rid of surface build-up. This means that anything sitting stubbornly on the surface of your skin, like dead cells and other debris, is dissolved.** They are mostly naturally occurring and are water soluble, meaning they can't get beneath the skin. They are excellent for getting rid of dead stuff, but also for evening out skin tone (by revealing new skin) and helping a bit with pigmentation and fine lines. Good on sun damage, too. Someone once explained it to me brilliantly like this: imagine your skin as a wall of bricks. The bricks are held together by mortar. Some of the mortar is old and crumbling, but kind of stuck on, giving the wall a sub-optimal, gnarly look. AHAs get rid of all the old, crumbly bits, so the wall becomes smooth and lovely. (This is a helpful metaphor, not a statement of fact. Your skin isn't going to look twenty-five again. But there will definitely be a significant improvement.) Some AHAs, like lactic and glycolic acids, are humectants too, which means they help with hydration. Use with caution on sensitive skin and do a patch test first.

- **Beta hydroxy acid, or BHA, gets rid of anything lurking deeper down. This means it goes some way into your pores and dissolves any build-up it finds in there. Salicylic acid is the BHA used in skincare.** It is oil soluble, meaning it can penetrate the natural oils on your skin and make its way down, and it has antibacterial and anti-inflammatory properties, so it's great, even transformative, for congested skin. It can also work wonders on rosacea.

Liquid exfoliants are as good as they sound – which is perhaps *too* good. They work so well and so quickly, and they're in so many different products these days, that the temptation is to overuse them and exist in a state of permanently renewing, refreshed skin. But don't do this. Overuse messes up your skin barrier, which is a terrible idea because the skin barrier's job is to keep moisture in (remember, it's all about moisture) and external aggressors, like pollution, out. It can also thin the skin barrier if used excessively over time, which is another thing you really don't want as this would accelerate signs of ageing. So, yes, they're great – but use cautiously. This is especially important if your beauty regime involves other 'actives', or products containing extremely effective active ingredients, like retinol, which we'll get to in a bit. It's your face – don't lob random ingredients at it just because you like the sound of what they can do. These ingredients are powerful.

How to use them

Gradually. Don't start with something massively strong – ease yourself in gently and your skin will thank you. Acids are in all sorts of products. I would start with a toner twice a week, or possibly a face wash (not both). It doesn't sound like much, but sit back and watch what happens. Important: they vary widely in strength, so always read the instructions that come with the product, and obey them – this is not an area where you want to go, 'I think I'll just use a bit extra.'

THE EDIT: SEVEN EXCELLENT LIQUID EXFOLIANTS

- **Biologique Recherche P50 (around £80)** has been around for decades – it's one of those 'why French women have good skin' products. (Probably. I hate those stupid books/articles that treat French women as a different species, with ploddy little British women gazing up in tragic adoration, saying, 'Show me how to be more like you.' It's borderline racist, actually, in both directions.) Now, there are lots of these products around, and at all sorts of prices. But this is turbo-charged. I don't recommend this particular one for reactive skin but there exist several excellent versions of P50, including one for sensitive skin. This one, though, is the *capo di tutti capi* of acid exfoliants. It contains polyacids, AHAs and BHA. There's also cider vinegar in there, and the product smells vinegary. You won't care. What it basically does is everything. It sloughs away dead skin and cells like a champ. It balances the pH surface of the skin. It kills blackheads and blemishes before they've even had a chance to form. And over time, it effectively gives you new skin, by getting rid of all the crap that's sitting on top of your current skin so that you wake up with a serious clear, smooth glow. It's brilliant and in my view is entirely worth its hefty price tag. Don't freestyle – read the leaflet and do what it tells you. Note: wear an SPF while you're using this.

- **Alpha H Liquid Gold (around £40)**. This is a glycolic acid treatment and possibly my all-time favourite skincare product. I know – it's some claim. But it gets rid of dead gubbins that's sitting there spoiling your face, it imparts marvellous radiance after just a few uses, it helps with fine lines and low levels of pigmentation *and* it hydrates beautifully – no need for a separate moisturizer. A multi-tasker as well as a wonder, and not insanely priced given how good it is. Use three times a week at the most. (You'll be so pleased with the results that you'll be tempted to do it more often. Don't).

- **Paula's Choice 2% BHA Exfoliant (around £34)** is brilliant for congested skin. I rate Paula's Choice products very highly generally too. Paula is Paula Begoun, who in 1992 wrote a fantastic book called *Don't Go to the Cosmetics Counter Without Me*, which fearlessly debunked many of the wild claims made by various brands about various products, dispassionately using science to prove or disprove the competence of hundreds of cosmetics. This eventually mutated into beautypedia.com, an extremely useful and recommended resource. She started her own brand in the mid-1990s. The products' packaging isn't necessarily going to win any design awards, but the contents are highly effective and contain no fragrances, dyes or other irritants.
- **Paula's Choice Skin Perfecting 8% AHA Gel Exfoliant (about £35), and Resist Anti-Ageing 10% AHA Exfoliant (around £39).** These aren't about excavating blocked pores but rather about addressing fine lines and wrinkles. They will also eventually fade brown spots – note: fade, not magically remove.
- **The Ordinary Glycolic Acid 7% Toning Solution (about £12).** Glycolic acid has the smallest molecule of the AHAs, so this gets in there fast and targets the signs of ageing. Good on uneven skin tone.

- **Pixi Glow Tonic (about £18)**. This was once wildly popular and deserves to be so again. People moved on to stronger solutions, but I think its 5% glycolic acid is a virtue – gentle enough not to traumatize but potent enough to be effective. A good one to start with, as is **REN's Ready Steady Glow Tonic (around £28)**.
- **Murad AHA/BHA Exfoliating Cleanser (about £43)** or **Murad Replenishing Multi-Acid Peel (about £70)**. Murad is another of my pet brands, because everything does what it says it will do. The cleanser is a good gateway drug if you'd rather wash the acid off before going to bed.

A serum is an extra skincare step that addresses specific concerns, like dark spots, fine lines, blotchiness or generally dull skin (though, frankly, dull skin shouldn't be a major issue if you exfoliate). They're oil- or water-based, slightly gloopy and highly concentrated, delivering a big old dose of their hero ingredient(s) to clean, prepped skin. They go on after cleansing but before moisturizing.

The question is, do you need one as well as a moisturizer? I thought for a long time that the answer was no, but I've done a massive U-turn and now think they're essential. The good ones are fantastic, and the closest skincare comes to miracles. Again, nothing short of cosmetic intervention will make you look ten years younger, but these are the ingredients that will make you look like the best version of yourself, which I think is a good place to head for.

Serums are often presented as quasi-magical potions, which they kind of are, an impression that is compounded by the fact that they come in serious-looking little bottles with droppers. They vary wildly in price, from under a tenner to hundreds of pounds. They vary wildly in efficacy, too, and price is not always a reliable indicator.

Let's try to break it down a bit. For simplicity's sake – this is where is gets techy and complicated very quickly – I'm going to stick to ingredients that I rate and don't think are in any way a con, rather than give you a giant list of every single one that exists. This is where things like retinols and peptides come in, so let's start there. I'll try to keep it super-simple.

- **Retinol** is vitamin A, or synthetic derivatives of vitamin A. Vitamin A encourages both skin renewal and collagen production. Collagen is a protein responsible for skin elasticity (and springy connective tissue, and thus healthy joints). Our production of it drops off in our thirties, hence wrinkles and sag. Vitamin A effectively glues itself to cells and instructs them to be pert and youthful, and – incredibly – they obey. It also combats free radicals (see Vitamin C below), which make skin look older, and is good at making pores *appear* smaller. It's pretty impressive. But not everyone can hack it – it's quite full-on and can be too irritating for some skins. You can use retinol with niacinamide. You can also use retinol with BHAs and AHAs, but it's a *lot*. I would personally exfoliate for a few weeks, then stop and go in with the retinol. Start with a product containing only a little (they go from 0.1% retinol to over 1%) and see how you get on before building up: as I was saying, it can be irritating. Don't think that a low percentage won't do much because it will.

- **Retinoids** are specific bits of vitamin A that have been split off from the vitamin A mothership. They are more powerful than the 'whole' vitamin A. You need a prescription for some of the stronger retinoids, like tretinoin, which is used in the treatment of acne.
- **Peptides** are amino acids and proteins. Collagen is made up of polypeptide chains. Peptides can penetrate the skin because they are small. The idea here is that adding them to skincare helps with collagen and can therefore improve elasticity and hydration as well as firm skin. You can use retinol and peptides together. I'd do peptides in the morning and retinol at night.
- **Vitamin C** is vitamin C, and I love it. It is a powerful antioxidant. (Donald Trump has spoiled the word 'powerful' for me, but never mind.) It's like a tiny superhero, particularly good at fighting free radicals, which are unstable molecules that are incomplete because they are missing electrons. They therefore roam the world seeking electrons to attach themselves to, like a band of bandits. Unfortunately, the process of attaching themselves causes damage to you, such as fine lines and wrinkles and other signs of ageing. But! Antioxidants, such as our

hero vitamin C, can attach themselves to the free radicals *before* said free rads can attach themselves to your nice healthy skin cells and, kerpow, they neutralize them. You know how if you're cooking you squeeze lemon juice over apples to stop them going brown? Same principle. You are the apple. Vitamin C is the lemon juice (in more ways than one).

It's not just signs of ageing. Because vitamin C is an antioxidant, it protects your skin from environmental damage. It can also help when it comes to UV damage manifesting as dark marks or hyper-pigmentation. If you use it regularly, it can even stop brown spots or dark marks appearing in the first place. (Allegedly. I already had brown spots when I started using it, so I can't personally vouch for that particular claim.) If the brown spots already exist, it can fade them without fading the rest of your skin. It will also help your sunscreen protect you better. These qualities also show themselves as an ability to even out and brighten skin tone generally – it's brilliant at this. Vitamin C will soften fine lines, blur acne scars, and restore brightness to skin that looks knackered. It's a really, really good thing to have on your shelf. It's unstable when exposed to light or air, and therefore comes appropriately packaged, often in dark glass.

You can use retinol and vitamin C together, though maybe not if you have sensitive skin. It's a powerful combo. Do one in the morning and one at night, keep a close eye on things and drop one if you start looking overly red or peely, bearing in mind that a degree of redness or peeliness can be part of the process.

- **Niacinamide** is vitamin B3. It is very good at tightening and reducing the appearance of large pores, at evening out skin tone, helping with dullness, softening fine lines and generally making the skin stronger and more resilient. It combats environmental damage and can at least partly reverse past damage of this kind; it's good on discoloration, including under-eye circles. Unusually, it plays well with others and you can use it in conjunction with any of these other super-ingredients. Niacinamide is a big deal because it is such an excellent multi-tasker and so well tolerated by skin.

- **Ceramides** are fats that exist naturally in your skin. Fats keep skin supple (obviously), but our ceramide quota depletes as we age, and with sun exposure. You can put them back in via ceramide-containing skincare. Synthetic ceramides can also 'teach' your skin to repair itself, which naturally derived ceramides can't do – a good example of natural not always being best. They're not stable when exposed to light and air, so they come in little plastic pods or in dark glass to keep them on an even keel. Good used around the eyes, too.

• **Hyaluronic acid** occurs naturally in skin. It is remarkable because it can hold on to a thousand times its weight in moisture. It's also a humectant, meaning it sucks in moisture from the outside world. Think bionic levels of hydration. Hyaluronic acid is great.

• **Azelaic acid**, which occurs naturally in various grains, is interesting. I'm including it in this list because it can be highly effective in treating mild to moderate acne, rosacea and pigmentation. The brand to investigate if that's you is Dermatica.

The easiest way of maximizing effectiveness when combining ingredients is by using a serum that does it all for you, which is where we came in.

Vitamin C serums

Everyone should have a vitamin C serum because they really work. Plus, unlike various other active products that really work, they probably won't freak your skin out for a bit when you start using them, unless your skin is extremely sensitive to begin with, in which case do a tiny patch test first.

If you want to splash out, then for me the king of vitamin C serums is **Skinceuticals's legendary C E Ferulic** (which is absolutely phenomenal but which costs **around £140**). If you want to really up the ante, you could combine a vitamin C serum with a clarifying acid toner. Here the high-end bee's knees is **Biologique Recherche's P50 (around £80)** (see p. 30) and its various relations, but again, it's expensive. Much cheaper versions include **Pixi's Glow Tonic (around £18)**.

THE EDIT: ELEVEN BRILLIANT SERUMS

- **La Roche-Posay Pure Retinol Serum (around £45)**. This contains normal retinol and gradual-release retinol, plus niacinamide and hyaluronic acid. Go for the same brand's **Retinol B3 Serum (around £45)** if you have sensitive skin.
- **Beauty Pie Super Retinol (around £16 for Beauty Pie members)**.* Contains retinol, lactic acid, hyaluronic acid and ceramides. A good all-rounder.

---

* Beauty Pie is an online-only brand to which you must have a subscription, currently costing about £10 a month. It's the brainchild of beauty expert Marcia Kilgore, who, among her many achievements, founded the Bliss Spa range (and FitFlops!). The idea is that they go to the very best scientists, labs, factories, etc., who create and manufacture world-class formulations – and then cut out the middlemen. This means they can lose the usual mark-ups (up to 70 per cent!) and offer customers seriously good products at wholly affordable prices. This strategy obviously rests entirely on how good the products are. I really rate them.

- **Medik8 Retinol 3TR (around £32)**. This is an excellent first retinol; you can eventually go on to the stronger 6TR version. Retinol, vitamin E and jojoba oil. Medik8 also make **Crystal Retinal Cream (around £45)**, which contains a next-generation retinol called retinaldehyde; you buy the product in increasing strengths. It works very fast. There's an eye cream version too.
- **Medik8 C-Tetra (around £40)**. A very good first vitamin C serum. You can graduate to **Medik8 C-Tetra Luxe**.
- **The Ordinary Granactive Retinoid 2% in Squalane (around £11)**. Less irritating than most due to its use of hydroxypinacolone retinoate, which is also supposed to work faster.
- **Sunday Riley Good Genes Glycolic Acid Treatment (around £70)**. This is a mighty serum that mainly works on unclogging pores, undoing sun damage, reducing fine lines and restoring elasticity. Smells weird. I really rate Sunday Riley as a brand, but I'm not sure anyone is buying it for its delicious scents. (I find this strangely reassuring – efficacy over 'pampering'.)
- **Beauty Pie Triple Hyaluronic Acid Lipopeptide Serum (around £19 for Beauty Pie members)**. Majorly hydrating for plumped, radiant skin. Not for you if you're oily; otherwise great.

- **Beauty Pie Youthbomb™ 360° Radiance Concentrate (around £44 to Beauty Pie members)**. This firms skin, adds radiance, hydrates and smooths the texture of the skin. As is usually the case with Beauty Pie, you get an awful lot of bang for your buck.
- **Institut Esthederm Age Proteom Advanced Serum (around £86)**. Developed for older skin. This protects against environmental aggressors, which age you like nobody's business. Leaves skin smoothed, toned and firm, or at least firmer.
- **Augustinus Bader The Retinol Serum (around £270)**. This is fantastic and worth it if you're very rich. This consistently impressive brand owns a patent for something called TFC8, a concoction of forty skincare ingredients designed to hurry along cell renewal. Here it is added to pure retinol.

As well as hydrating, moisturizer soothes. Say you've been swimming in the sea on a sunny day: even if you don't hold with serums, exfoliants and the like, and even if your skincare routine simply consists of washing your face in Fairy Liquid,* it is a fact that applying a thin layer of whatever cream or lotion you have to hand when you get home after your swim will make your face feel a great deal more comfortable. If you *have* been using all or any of the acids and serums above, their very effectiveness makes them startling, sometimes even shocking, to skin, which benefits afterwards from the equivalent of being wrapped up in a nice cosy blanky and given a soothing drink, i.e. being moisturized.

Of course not all moisturizers are created equal – but this is another area where prices sometimes differ by hundreds of pounds. (I must digress here and answer one of the questions I'm asked most often, which is: *Is Crème de la Mer*† *worth it?* Short answer: kind of, if you're

* Fairy Liquid is the only thing that will remove disastrous box hair dye. It will also leave your hair like straw, but you can't have everything.
† Crème de la Mer was invented by a Dr Max Huber to treat his own burns – he was an astrophysicist in the 1950s. The story sounds a bit sketchy, largely because there is no online obituary for him, but US *Elle*

fifty plus, have fine lines, dry to very dry skin and can afford it. It is hyper-rich – too rich, in my view, for younger skin, for skin that isn't gasping for hydration, and for oilier skins. Some might find it too rich to use in warm weather too – it's like solidified clotted cream. But, yes, it will turn your dry or very dry skin to smooth, bright, even loveliness. Its trademarked Miracle Broth, apparently invented to heal the founder's burns, involves fermented seaweed extracts. It's not the only thing that does, though.

I feel I've banged on enough about the importance of keeping skin supple, and how it's your best defence against premature ageing, but I'll just say it one more time for emphasis. Supple skin feels – and looks – full of life and vitality. It is comfortable, plump and well fed, not tight and slightly caved-in-looking. Makeup sits well on top of it. By contrast, dehydrated skin feels tight, maybe itchy, perhaps even painful, and makeup perches stubbornly above the dryness of it, refusing to meld or blend. Like anything left to dry out, dehydrated skin acquires lines and loses plumpness. Since our ageing

---

magazine dug down and, yes, he did exist – he worked for an aerospace company called Cal-Val, not for NASA as is widely reported. *Elle* interviewed an Austrian countess (obviously) who met him – 'He was very tall and had the skin of a twelve-year-old' – and was instrumental in making the cream a word-of-mouth sensation in the US. There are photographs. Anyway, it was the first very expensive face cream, though it's been overtaken on that front and then some. Many people absolutely swear by it.

dermis is doing both those things all by itself anyway, it seems silly to compound the issue by not at least attempting to compensate for what is being lost.

Now, I believe that most moisturizers are quite good, even when they're 99p. I know, heresy! Remember what I was saying about differences in price often being largely down to packaging? That's very much the case here. No doubt some actively terrible moisturizers exist, and certainly some are so packed with artificial fragrance that just sniffing them gives you a rash, but in years of testing stuff I haven't come across one that I wanted to chuck across the room in disgust: in terms of moisturizing, they all work to a greater or lesser extent. If you're looking to save money, my advice is: invest in a brilliant serum and buy a cheaper moisturizer.

I say this confidently because the whole concept of moisturizers is really simple. Moisturizers have one job, which is to add a bit of moisture – water – to your skin, and then to trap it in, which they do by being oily/greasy, or nourishing/rich to put it more attractively. As well as water, which is always the main ingredient, moisturizers also contain:

- humectants, which draw water from the air and (up to a point) from the deeper layers of the skin. They're not much cop when the air is dry, so they need . . .
- occlusives, which provide the gloop that traps the water. Petrolatum is the best at holding in

water – it's also known as petroleum jelly, a.k.a. Vaseline. So why not use Vaseline? you reasonably ask. Because it's too greasy and liable to break you out in spots, unfortunately – though by all means try it if you're extremely dry. Other water-trappers might be fatty alcohols, lanolin (the grease on sheep wool), lecithin, paraffin, mineral oil and stearic acid, or silicones like dimethicone.

- emollients, which make skin feel smooth.
- certain vitamins, which, as we saw on page 40, can make a big difference if they are in a format in which their molecules are stable. That format isn't usually reliably usable in moisturizers – but it is in serums.

Now, of course some moisturizers also contain much fancier and more advanced skincare ingredients than others; some smell nicer; some have a more luxurious texture and absorb better; and some make a point of specifically addressing certain signs of ageing, though since we're trying to address loss of elasticity through lack of hydration, even a basic moisturizer is going to help. The main thing is matching your moisturizer to your skin type, so that it does enough but doesn't overwhelm – or, in other words, so it doesn't clog your skin. Having said all that, here are some of my favourites. Remember that you pay for packaging.

THE EDIT: SEVEN GREAT MOISTURIZERS

- **Weleda Skin Food Nourishing Day Cream (around £15)** – there's also a night cream. I have loved Weleda Skin Food since the days when you could only get it in grungy hippie health-food shops that smelt of incense. The body lotion is a fantastic moisturizer, plus it smells divine. Packed with botanical extracts, the newer day and night creams are just as fabulous.
- One of my favourite high-end brands is **MZ Skin**, this being the brainchild of Dr Maryam Zamani. Her products came passionately recommended by someone whose judgement I trust, and she wasn't wrong. I point you to one of two moisturizers, one rich, **The Rich Moisturizer (around £150)** and one light (guess), either of which someone older – like, middle-aged to ancient – would be delighted to receive. I am convinced that the light one made my skin firmer when I tested it, and the rich one contains bio-identical human collagen, which claims not just to firm and smooth but to actually lift. On the basis of these and of the excellent **Placenta* and Stem Cell Night**

---

* I know, placenta, ew. And also ewe: it is ovine placenta, so from sheep rather than from humans. If you don't want to rob a bank in order to

Serum (around £235) – Dr Maryam is not mucking about – I would happily recommend anything from the range. Ditto that by **Dr David Jack** – super-simple, super-effective (see p. 96n)

- I also very much rate the fabulously bluntly named **Shiseido Benefiance Wrinkle Smoothing Cream (around £87)**. It contains what the brand calls ReNeura technology, which basically shouts at your skin to sort itself out. I saw a clear and distinct improvement in fine lines within three weeks. The older friend I gave a pot to for Christmas two years ago has still not stopped raving about it.
- **Elemis Pro-Collagen Marine Cream (around £95)**. Like La Mer (see page 49), Elemis have their own marine extract, present in this specifically anti-ageing cream. Using it makes a visible difference to my skin – it is plumper, juicier, smoother. Their independent clinical trials say that usage 'reduces the appearance of wrinkle depth by up to 78%' – I wouldn't necessarily go that far but I really believe in this cream. Try to get about two weeks' worth of samples before coughing up – you should see a difference in that time.

---

afford to put sheep placenta on your face, that's okay and I hear ya. There are many other options. But it is an outstanding serum.

- **La Roche-Posay Toleriane Sensitive Moisturizer (around £14)** is excellent on redness and irritation, or when your skin feels stressed and tight. No irritants, plus ceramides. La Roche-Posay is an outstanding brand and I rate their (very many, concern-specific) other moisturizers too.
- **Vichy Minéral 89 Moisture Boosting Cream (around £22)**. Hyaluronic acid aplenty, plus squalane to boost. Nice fresh texture, feels great on the skin, absorbs instantly. Has obsessive devotees.
- **Curél Intensive Moisture Facial Cream (around £20)**. This is a great, simple – but not that simple: the brand is Japanese and the cream contains a clever pseudo-ceramide – moisturizer that would suit most people with normal to dry skin (including sensitive) very nicely indeed. The very definition of 'You don't need to spend a fortune on your moisturizer.'

I like to seal in moisturizer with facial oil. Not all year round – this isn't something I'd do in summer or if I was somewhere boiling hot. But in winter, when my skin is given to feeling parched because of the contrast between central heating and cold weather, I recommend it, unless your skin is already oily, in which case it might be too much. Try one, though – my skin is combination and I get on with them marvellously. You're trying to seal in moisture using something fatty: oils cut to the chase. You're trying to lubricate your skin and make it supple: oils do that. What they can't do is penetrate very deeply, because their molecules are too big. But if moisturizer is the blanket, oil is the eiderdown. Press oil in with your fingers rather than rubbing it in like cream.

THE EDIT: THREE FAVOURITE FACE OILS

- **Votary's Super Boost Night Drops (around £95)**. Thrillingly, said drops contain CBD oil. I'm sent tons of products with CBD oil and never really understand what it does. I sniff them all to see if they smell of weed, but they never do, which I find obscurely disappointing. Anyway – now I know. CBD oil, according to Votary, has quasi-magical properties when it comes to soothing irritation and redness, and calming 'the skin's mantle' (any brand that mentions 'the skin's mantle' is all right with me). It also reduces sebum production, which is good if you're oily, and it restores elasticity if you're aged. Here it is mixed with strawberry-, flax-, camellia-, poppy- and sunflower-seed oils and rosemary leaf extract. What I really like about it – I'm always slightly wary of oils in case they make me look like a used frying pan – is that it sinks in instantly. I thought my skin was perfectly well hydrated, but if it were a cartoon it would have gone GULP and asked

for more. There was no oily residue whatsoever.
If I didn't know better, I'd think I'd been using the
wrong moisturizer, but I haven't. Pop on a few
drops at night for a little while, and move on to
adding a drop to your normal night cream or
moisturizer. Your skin will thank you. I rate this
brand generally: the cleansing oils are gorgeous to
use and get every last scrap of makeup off and the
**Intense Night Oil with rosehip and retinoid
(around £135)** is a genuine skin-saver in times of
desperate need, to say nothing of **Super Seed
Facial Oil (around £70)**.

- **de Mamiel's Winter Facial Oil (around
  £85)** – they do four seasonal ones each year.
  These oils are organic, ECOCERT certified
  and absolutely packed with goodness. The
  Winter version includes a ton of helpful stuff,
  from argan and marula oils to soften and plump,
  to oils that encourage collagen production, skin
  renewal, protection from free radicals, and so
  on. All you really need to know, though, is that I
  put this on my face before bed and my skin
  drank it in: it was like giving it a present. The
  price is worth paying if you can afford it. If your
  skin is feeling dry, slightly withered, lacklustre,
  flat, dreary, un-radiant and generally under par,
  it will sort it out and calm it down without any
  mysterious or questionable ingredients. Note:
  it's fine on oily skin – just don't slather it on.

- **Alexandra Soveral** is a fantastic London-based facialist (see alexandrasoveral.co.uk), who uses natural products and her hands rather than anything spookier. The results are immediately visible. She also does outstanding face oils, which you can buy through her website. I use and love **Forever Young (around £50)**, which contains antioxidants, fatty acids and natural essential oils.

A NOTE ON LUXURY PRODUCTS

Whenever I recommend something expensive, I am reminded of the late Diana Vreeland's legendary advice column in *Harper's Bazaar*. Vreeland eventually became the magazine's fashion editor and went on to edit US *Vogue*, where she had her office walls painted in scarlet lacquer and sent memos to staff saying things like 'Today let's think pig white! Wouldn't it be wonderful to have stockings that were pig white! The color of baby pigs, not quite white and not quite pink!' I really love Diana Vreeland (there was a marvellous autobiography called *D.V.*, now sadly out of print but available second-hand from the usual places). When she died in 1989, the great photographer Richard Avedon said, 'She was and remains the only genius fashion editor.'

It all started in 1936, when she was offered a job at *Harper's Bazaar* by its editor, Carmel Snow, who went up to her after she'd seen her dancing at a club wearing a white Chanel lace dress and roses in her hair. Vreeland said, 'But Mrs Snow, I've never worked. I've never been in an office in my life. I'm never dressed until lunch.' This wasn't considered an issue, and before long Vreeland was making helpful suggestions in her column 'Why Don't You?': 'Why don't you . . . rinse your blond child's hair in dead champagne to keep it gold, as they do in France?' was one, along with 'Why don't you . . . have an elk-hide trunk for the back of your car? Hermès of Paris will make this.' I wonder if she made herself laugh thinking them up. My feeling is very much not.

THE EDIT: FOUR OTHER EXCELLENT
FACE OILS (that won't all break the bank)

- **Sunday Riley Luna Sleeping Night Oil (around £45).** This has retinol in it as well as botanicals. It is extremely effective, particularly on older skin and/or on rosacea, acne, eczema and other woes.
- **Sunday Riley CEO Glow (around £65).** The glow, which is very real, comes from vitamin C (see page 39). If you want radiance, this is your guy. Well, one of them.
- **The Ordinary 100% Organic Cold Pressed Rosehip Seed Oil (around £10).** Quite sticky,

but if you're just looking for something to seal your cream in, it does the job perfectly.

- **Biossance 100% Squalane Oil (around £26)**. Squalane with an *a* mimics squalene with an *e*, this being a lipid that we produce naturally until, you've guessed it, we stop producing it quite so effectively as we age. It also exists in things like olives and sugarcane, but not in a usable format – it goes rancid too fast. So it is hydrogenated, and lo, squalane. The goodness of this oil is that you can use it everywhere, including on your face, body and on dried-out hair ends. You only need a very little. I find squalane oil highly effective and an excellent bargain.

You should feel quite pleased to have oily skin. I know it can be a pain, but the thing to remember is that it is resilient and doesn't age nearly as quickly as non-oily skin. Give yourself a gold star. As for *spot*-spots, as opposed to occasional spots: leaving aside diet – which makes a *huge* difference to skin,* as does being sufficiently hydrated – I don't feel qualified to give advice on serious adult acne. For anything not quite serious, but annoying enough to be an issue, I refer you to some of the acids and serums on pages 42–5 and to Sunday Riley's Luna face oil (see page 59). BHAs (beta hydroxy acids, see page 29) are designed to get deep into the pores and zap any excess sebum or debris, so they're a very good place to start. Please don't be tempted to go from zero to nuclear by using the highest strengths and the most powerful products from the outset. They will traumatize your skin, which is perfectly likely to produce *more* oil in response to being stripped of it. It's also likely to become inflamed.

* I'm obviously not a dietician, but you can find one online by checking with the Association of British Dieticians, who keep a directory of accredited professionals who meet their high standards.

Now, sometimes I come across a product that makes me want to race around clanging a bell and shouting, 'Oyez, oyez!' at the top of my lungs, red in the face with exertion. This is such a product. What we have here is nothing short of miraculously effective for spots, acne-prone and congested skin. And get this – you can see a really dramatic difference inside forty-eight hours, and by dramatic I mean DRAMATIC. I could hardly believe my eyes. Nor could anyone else – when I tested this on my teenage guinea pig, the improvement was so quick and striking that everyone in the house remarked on it. You couldn't fail to notice. 'Oh, my God,' said one. 'That's incredible. What on earth are you using?'

Bioderma's new **Sebium Kerato+** cream, is the answer, morning and night, in conjunction with their foaming **Sebium Actif gel wash (around £13)** rinsed off with a clean hot flannel. (I like this non-drying gel wash a lot. It feels almost like an oil and is a brilliant cleanser for problem skin.) What we have here are spot-destroying keratolytic acids, namely 10 per cent malic acid ester (the 'ester' bit means this new-generation AHA works *with* the pH of your skin rather than blasting it willy-nilly) and 1.8 per cent salicylic acid, a BHA that dissolves the keratin in dead skin cells and therefore allows the sebum to escape normally, rather than to sit there trapped and turning itself into a blackhead or worse out of sheer rage (I imagine). The result is soft, smooth, hydrated skin, with a noticeable improvement in existing marks.

It isn't just the crazy speed with which this cream works that impressed me so much. What is so good about this product is that it doesn't dry anything out. We're all familiar with spot treatments that basically nuke the skin, to the point where the spot is so dried up that it is forced to die. That's fine, but it gives you horrible skin, tight and peely, red in places, sore-looking, irritated, sensitized. This genius cream doesn't do that. The spot dies, but the skin on and around it remains soft and hydrated – *ergo*, no discomfort, redness, peeling or anything else. Skin looks alive and skin-like, not withered and traumatized.

As I've said at least a dozen times over the years, I love Bioderma, who make outstanding, affordable skincare for everyone, whatever their skin concern. They don't have a duff product in their entire range, but this one is really the cherry on the cake. It's the best spots – I'm using the plural even though it looks weird because this is about much more than the odd isolated blemish – treatment I've ever come across, the kind of product I feel quite moved by, because it'll free squillions of people from the tyranny of bad skin. It's genius.

I suppose I should probably add that I only tried it on acne-prone skin, rather than acne-acne skin, but put it this way: on Day 1 there were more spots and blemishes than clear skin – dozens of them – and by Day 6 every single one had either gone or faded to near-invisibility.

THE EDIT: EIGHT REALLY GOOD BRANDS
FOR SPOT-PRONE MATURE SKIN*

- **Bioderma**, as above.
- **La Roche-Posay's Effaclar** range.
- **CeraVe**'s range for oily skin.
- **Paula's Choice**, various, but the **Skin Perfecting 2% BHA Liquid Exfoliant (around £34)** makes a lot of formerly spotty people rave with gratitude.
- **Starface face stickers (around £12)** – these contain salicylic acid, which is a BHA, as well as hydrocolloid, which flattens by absorbing bacteria and gunk. You stick them on the more hideous spots and leave them to do their job. Yes, they're star-shaped, but I like that about them. Note: they're for big old spots with a head, not for headless skin bumps. Headless skin bumps are the worst. Use a BHA like the Paula's Choice one above on those.
- **Murad**'s range for spots and blemishes, in particular their **Jumbo InvisiScar Resurfacing Treatment (around £38)**, which is excellent at minimizing post-spot scarring, hyper-pigmentation (though see also pages 40 and 77) and general dark marks.

* See page 153 for the best concealers.

- As I was saying earlier, azelaic acid is very effective on mild to moderate acne. If that's you, have a look at **Dermatica (from about £20)**. It also works on rosacea and hyper-pigmentation.
- You'll need a really good oil-free sunscreen and my recommendation is for **Heliocare's Oil-Free Gel (around £30),** which is light, packed with antioxidants, has SPF50 and is mattifying.

Possibly the most important line in this whole skincare section: it is estimated that at least 80 per cent of the signs of ageing are caused by sun damage. The United States Environmental Protection Agency, an official website of the US Government, put the figure at 90 per cent. All those fine lines don't just appear out of thin air because you've hit a milestone birthday. Of course skin withers as we age and as production of all the helpful things that have kept it perky in its youth slows down. But the sun accelerates the withering to a crazy extent. As well as lines, we develop sun spots: years of exposure to UV light causes melanin, the pigment in our skin, to be produced in excess amounts. Those dark marks starts appearing where the sun most hits us, so on faces, hands, forearms and upper chests.*

This is why everyone constantly bangs on about always wearing sun protection. We all know this, but it's worth reiterating. So is the unavoidable fact that you need to reapply sun protection throughout the day. Here I think a lot of people do less well – because it's a faff, because we forget, because we've done our makeup and don't want to

* Also, skin cancer.

smear sunscreen about on top of it (see page 73), or possibly because we remember sunscreen from when we had small children: it was so white and dense that it made them look like little ghosts, and now we think we'll wear a big hat, stay in the shade and take our chances.

Things have moved on from the ghost-children days, so let me recommend some undetectable, ungreasy, user-friendly, dedicated sunscreens that feel nice on the skin before we get into what we can (and can't) do about sun spots, brown spots, call them what you will, and about sun-inflicted lines.

A quick reminder:

- UVA rays are longer, and cause damage deeper down. UBV rays are shorter, and damage the surface of the skin, as well as causing burning. UVA rays can travel through glass, including that of your car windscreen or sunny office. About 95 per cent of the solar radiation that reaches the Earth is UVA.
- There are two kinds of sunscreen: chemical and mineral. Chemical sunscreens soak up the rays, as if they were tiny sponges. Mineral sunscreens deflect them, as if they were Captain America's shield, so they bounce off. Chemical filters are absorbed by the skin, meaning no ghostliness. Mineral filters sit on top. Chemical filters don't always agree with people with very sensitive skin, plus their chemicals leach into the sea

when you go swimming – they're banned in some places, usually where there are coral reefs. It's up to you: that needn't necessarily be an issue when you're sitting in the office. I tend to favour mineral filters.

• Remember to take your sun protection right down to the tops of your cleavage if you are on a beach or wearing something strapless. Sun damage on the chest is hard to fix.

SPF sprays

A lot of people find the combination of makeup and sunscreen a bit of a faff, not least because of fear of pore blockage. Makes sense: it's hot, your skin gets hot, and the last thing you want is layers of products clogging everything up and melting slightly at the same time. It's an unappetizing recipe.

Nevertheless, I still wear sunscreen as a base layer, with makeup on top. This is good, and I recommend everyone does it, but there is one obvious problem: sunscreen, as I've said above, needs reapplication throughout the day. It's not an issue if you're on a beach, or barefaced, but if you're wearing any kind of makeup on your skin, it's a massive bummer. What are you supposed to do? Take everything off in the loos at work and start again from scratch, which is both time-consuming and wasteful, or reapply the sunscreen on top of the makeup, thereby risking a horrible smeary sort of soup?

You need an SPF spray. More, you need an SPF spray that sets makeup and has a slight but flattering blurring effect, that feels lovely and cool on the face, and that smells nice. This exists as a product by Kate Somerville, who used to be the beauty editor of the *Daily Telegraph*: **UncompliKated SPF Soft Focus Makeup Setting Spray (around £36)**. I love this product. It sat around for a bit before I tried it because I'm wary of things that sound a bit like hairspray for the face, even though they work very well and are, I would imagine, invaluable if you're spending the summer clubbing in Ibiza. (Do older people still spend the summer clubbing in Ibiza? I hope so.)

This spray is not those sprays. It's a more refined, elegant even, creation and, crucially, contains SPF 50 sunscreen. It doesn't feel sticky to use – on the contrary, it is super-refreshing, and scented with the zingy-but-becalming lavender essential oil. It's such a good idea – it takes two seconds to use, sets your makeup and stops you looking too shiny, and protects you from sun damage (though not all day – as with all sunscreens, you need to reapply every couple of hours). It contains hyaluronic acid for hydration and smoothness, and light-diffusing silicone powder to blur and soften things a bit. It reminds me of those big cans of Evian that my stepmother used to spray on her face all summer long, except that as well as feeling cooling and refreshing, this actually does important work too. Don't use it as your main sunscreen, obviously – it would work out hideously expensive. Instead, use it whenever you suspect your normal sunscreen could do with a top-up, or if you're unexpectedly still in the sun because it's such a beautiful afternoon, or because you're boiling and feel like your makeup is melting. It's not cheap, but all that you need is the finest, sheerest mist. Matte finish. This is a chemical sunscreen.

The high-street version, also recommended, is **Garnier Ambre Solaire Over Makeup Super UV Protection Mist SPF50 (around £12).** Like UncompliKated, you just spritz this on over your makeup. Also contains hyaluronic acid. The finish is dewy. (Also a chemical sunscreen.)

THE EDIT: FOUR REALLY GOOD SUNSCREEN BRANDS

- **Heliocare**. This is one that dermatologists recommend. Technologically and scientifically on the button. Protects against UVA, UVB, VL and IR rays, neutralizes free radicals and seeks to repair sun damage from the inside while preventing it happening on the outside. Not the cheapest, but worth it: I use **Heliocare 360 Oil-Free Gel (around £31)** as a daily sunscreen and swear by it. Mineral.
- **La Roche-Posay Anthelios**. Also dermatologist-recommended. I use **Anthelios Age Correct (around £25)**: it is particularly

recommended, but the whole range is excellent and covers all sorts of specific needs. The most recent iteration is **Anthelios UVmune 400 Invisible Fluid SPF50+ Sunscreen (around £20)**, which contains their own ingredient called Mexoryl 400 to protect against long UVA rays. Their research shows that these do even deeper damage than standard UVAs and UVBs. Yay. Mineral.

- **Garnier Ambre Solaire Super UV Anti Dark Spots & Anti Pollution Face Fluid SPF50 (around £8)**. Quite skincare-like, and contains hyaluronic acid. Feels exceptionally light on the skin. Chemical.
- **Vichy Capital Soleil Solar Protective Water Hydrating SPF50 (around £19.50)**. As its name suggests, this is water-like. Again with hyaluronic acid, so is highly hydrating. Chemical.

Dealing with sun damage

What can you realistically do about sun damage? The honest answer is, only a little – though not nothing! – by using products you apply to the skin, and quite a lot – though not everything! – if you're happy, and can afford, to ramp things up enough to enter the world of 'tweakments' (see page 83). This is because while superficial damage can be addressed up to a point with topical products, anything deeper – like the damage wrought by decades' worth of exposure to UVA rays – is unreachable. Creams simply can't penetrate deep enough. That kind of damage needs the big guns.

Skincare

First things first: many of the products that can help with sun damage also make your skin extra-sensitive to more sun damage. If you're going to use them, you need to be fanatical about sun protection. For this reason, I personally do not use them in summer (in the UK) and I would only ever use them at night. I'd still wear sunscreen in the daytime, even in winter. UVA rays are there doing their thing even when it's cloudy.

Now. Skincare can do a number of things. It can improve elasticity, improve the function of your skin's barrier, improve – but not get rid of – hyper-pigmentation and improve fine lines.

We covered the ingredients that help in Serums (pages 38–42), but as a reminder they are:

1. Niacinamide, which has many virtues (see page 41), including being good at fading dark marks. I have recommended several products already, but if you need more, try **SkinCeuticals Metacell Renewal B3 cream (around £100)**. Niacinamide is vitamin B3 and this cream is specifically formulated to speed up cell turnover and reduce the look of dark marks. SkinCeuticals is one of my favourite

'medical' brands. They are right at the forefront of new things that work.

2. Retinols (see page 38). These are vitamin A and speed up cell turnover, as well as being good on fine lines, improving the texture of the skin and working to fade hyper-pigmentation.

3. Vitamin C (see page 39). Good for repairing skin damage that's already taken place and, because it neutralizes free radicals, good at helping to prevent future damage too.

4. AHAs (see page 28) work at reducing skin pigmentation. Use at night.

The bigger guns – more serious but non-surgical options

Lasers

What can lasers do for sun damage? They can reach it, for starters, because they penetrate deep into the skin. They are also very good at smoothing the texture of the skin, so that it looks less like a linen sheet and more like something hotel-like and ironed. They generally do this by basically freaking your skin out so that it starts healing itself by upping its production of collagen. In the case of sun damage, the laser targets melanin, i.e. brown spots, and effectively blasts the relevant pigment cells to smithereens. These are then excreted. (The same principle applies with red skin, like thread veins, which lasers are good at getting rid of: they target haemaglobin instead of melanin.)

IPL

Lasers are the big-gun, non-surgical option. IPL, intense pulsed light, is cheaper and less invasive. It's also used for hair removal (see page 109) but is good at other things too, including age spots, which it addresses in pretty much the same way as lasers: the IPL makes a beeline for the melanin that is making the brown marks and breaks it up; it is then excreted by the body. Unless you have white skin and no tan, be cautious with IPL – it can get confused when it encounters darker skin and make matters worse. The brown spots may return after a while, in which case you can have them zapped again.

Lasers and IPLs are the best, most realistic options for sun spots (I'll get to lines in Tweakments, pages 83–94), and some people swear by them, especially lasers, which do absolutely improve skin texture and tautness. But both laser treatment and IPL can go wrong. They may *cause* hyper-pigmentation, which is the opposite of the desired effect. Approach with caution.

Brown and Black Skin

While I have seen lasers work well for sun spots on many people, I have seen catastrophic results on others (well, two others, but one would have been enough).

For a long time, lasers didn't really work on skin that

wasn't white, as in Caucasian. Then time passed, things evolved, and practitioners touted the greatness of their new brown-skin-friendly lasers. But the two people I know for whom lasers didn't work had brown skin. Long story short: instead of fading existing marks, the lasers triggered the production of more melanin, causing more dark brown marks.

I do know other brown-skinned people who've had effective laser treatment, though for tightening rather than fading purposes. I'm not claiming it doesn't work on a lot of people, but it's quite the risk, isn't it, lasering your face and wondering what will happen next? Which is why, having dark skin, I've never had it done.

On top of that, the people who sell these incredibly powerful machines sometimes train aestheticians for a matter of hours. If you're going to have laser or any kind of invasive treatment, it is absolutely imperative that you go to someone excellent and overqualified, like a medical doctor who specializes in aesthetics. I can't say it enough: this is not the time to hunt around for a bargain. Years ago a friend was bored and, walking past a chiropodist somewhere at the seaside, noticed they were also offering tattooed brows and eyeliner at bargain basement prices. She went in and had it done, like a lunatic. The liner wasn't too bad but the eyebrows were comedy-level awful and took years to fade. People laugh at this story and shake their heads in disbelief, but many are doing a version of exactly the same thing by going for cheap 'tweakments'. This isn't where you economize!

If you really want them and can't afford them, save up until you can see a properly qualified person. Anything else is playing roulette with your face.

Having said all that, if you have brown or Black skin and are at least laser-curious, I would suggest going to see a brown- or Black-skinned dermatologist offering these treatments. This is not my area of expertise but at the 2023 *Sunday Times* Style Beauty awards, the winner of the Skin Industry Expert category was London-based Dr Ewoma Ukeleghe, who has an active presence on social media, where she discusses these matters in detail.

For more on tweakments – what they are, what they're good for, who to go to, and so on – read on.

PART 1
Skincare

I'm conflicted about tweakments, treatments, work, non-surgical interventions, call them what you will. I fundamentally dislike the idea of having stuff injected into your face, or of having your face zapped or rollered or hoicked, all in a doomed, futile and perhaps even slightly deranged attempt at recapturing lost youth. I don't like the sentiment behind it, which is the opposite of acceptance. This is a problem, because for me the issue of ageing with a modicum of grace hinges around acceptance – of yourself, your looks, your flaws, skin biology and gravity.

I don't like the excuses people make for tweakments, or how they seek to normalize them. I find the idea that 'It's feminist if I say it is' – a convenient piece of nonsense much put about in the past decade and applied to everything from sex work to injectables – completely absurd. Wishing something were true doesn't make it so, and it doesn't strike me as particularly feminist to spend hundreds or thousands of pounds on looking 'better' than your contemporaries – on cheating, if you were being really condemnatory about it. I also find silly (and dangerous) the idea that tweakments are totally normal by virtue of high-profile people talking about them breezily – 'I have it done, therefore it's fine, it's nothing.' Maybe, but it's less likely to be so for someone younger and poorer with no access to a reputable practitioner. Mainly, though, there's a kind of vanity I strongly don't like, and tweakments are at its border.

But the border is porous. I also don't like judging women for their choices, whether those choices are rinsing your face in morning dew and calling it a day or having a face full of tweaks. And I can see – or, rather, I can't see – how good, even brilliant, some of the work is. I can't pin it down without asking. All I can see is someone looking fantastic in the most unobvious way, and when I finally winkle it out of them, I always briefly wonder whether I should have the same procedure myself. I always make a note of the doctor's name. I particularly appreciate older faces that look very natural – fresh, un-made-up, or as close to un-made-up as it gets (less always being more in this age group, as we'll see in Part 2: Makeup) – and those faces most often belong to either the genetically super-blessed or to people who have had very good work. The fact remains: one of my jobs is writing about beauty, which gives me access to all the free tweakments my heart could possibly desire. And yet here I am, entirely natural of face. Although . . . Well, read on.

Face cowboys

I'm just going to say it again: this whole area is shamefully under-regulated. It is terrifyingly easy to 'qualify' as a person with a big syringe who injects God knows what into God knows where. If I went on a course tomorrow, I could frame my certificate, buy myself a white coat and set up a couple of days later, perfectly legally, gaily injecting toxins and other substances into random people to my heart's content. I could give you fillers (and the rest) that would live in your face, wherever I'd seen fit to put them, for up to eighteen months.

Of course, there are highly reputable people who are highly skilled at doing this work, who are true artists – and having a good eye for composition should be a prerequisite. Their expertise can be transformative in the best possible way. But they are the exceptions, and you really need to do your homework finding them. Don't ever base your decision on cost. Good people are not cheap. It's annoying, but there we are: facts is facts. Don't base your decision on geographical proximity either – yes, it *is* amazingly convenient to find someone who does this stuff two streets away, or in your local salon, or who'll come to the house, but we both know that this person is unlikely to be the virtuoso you're looking for. Accept from the outset that you'll probably have to travel.

Do also base your decision on personal recommendations (this is really the best way), on having a really good look at the people making them, on having a consultation first, and on taking your research very seriously. I would always recommend seeing a qualified medical doctor, ideally someone whose training has included specialist knowledge of facial musculature, though I wouldn't automatically discount their nurse if she or he had been working alongside the doctor for a long time.

Do base your decision on what your prospective practitioner looks like. This is their job: they are their own best advertisement. Do they look weird? If so, they're not for you, unless you, too, want to look weird. Do they look like they've had too much done? Ditto. It's very easy to persuade yourself that your practitioner looks slightly OTT only because they're trying everything out on themselves, or that they 'have' to look that way because of their job. They would be much lighter-handed and subtler on you, you think, if you asked them to be. Actually, they wouldn't. They look how they look because they feel they look great. And good for them! Everyone's allowed the aesthetic they like. But if your idea of great clearly doesn't correspond to theirs, they're not the person for you.

For the same reason, have a look at the other people in the waiting room. (In certain London practices you will eventually spot at least one well-known older woman who is celebrated for ageing naturally.*) And never be too embarrassed to ask the practitioner for testimonials or photographs. A strange thing happens whenever British people find themselves in any kind of vaguely medical

---

* I really wish people wouldn't do this. It's like saying you keep yourself fit running about after the children when in fact you have three nannies.

situation: they tend to become passive, over-polite, over-worried about asking 'stupid' questions, and frightened of being 'annoying'. There are no stupid questions. It's your face. Be as annoying as you like. Make a list of everything you'd like to know, no matter how basic, and ask away. If you're not satisfied with the replies, or if the person gets shirty or patronizing, don't use them.

Aside from finding the best practitioner possible, the best piece of advice about tweakments that I can give you is this: **replace what was there before. Don't try to add what never existed.** Stick to this rule, don't overdo it, and you are unlikely to emerge looking troubling.

Injectables and me (Part One)

I have had Botox and fillers in the past, though (prior to writing this book) not for six or seven years, including one bad lot that made me look unignorably Neanderthal around the brow and eyes. That was a one-off (possibly a two-off, actually – I've tried to blank them out). But the good ones were good: I wrote at the time about how marvellous it was no longer to have a frown line between my eyebrows, and how my marionette lines – the unlovely name for the lines that go from the corners of your mouth to your chin – had been pleasingly softened.

These lines have all been back for years, deeper and more present. They have been joined by new ones. They don't drive me to despair, but I don't love them. I don't feel delighted to have them. I'm not 'proud' of them, as some young people seem to believe older people should be when it comes to all and any wrinkles. Being proud of your C-section scar is one thing, or of the deep lines of frowning concentration you have acquired from reading so much, squinting at weighty tomes or maybe exciting formulae long into the night. But proud of your sun damage? Duty-bound to let your face tell the story of your long and unfortunate relationship with sunbeds in the 1980s and 1990s? I understand the sentiment behind the calls for pride: of course our life's stories are written in our faces and bodies, and of course it would be madness to seek to erase them all. But that doesn't mean all the stories are worth telling.

Still, my lines don't cause me excessive distress. I have a fat face, which has the one great advantage of meaning that I am, in my own mind at least, fairly unlined. I also have relatively oily skin, which helps. I might feel much less ambivalent about this whole topic if my skin was more *obviously* wrinkled, or *clearly* thinning, or *covered* with brown spots, or actively leathery, or if I were just a few years older than I am, of the generation that anointed themselves with SPF0 oil and roasted themselves in the sun under one of those silver reflective three-part mirror things, and now have the severe sun damage to prove it. Or if I still lived in London and was endlessly comparing my face to those of fully tweaked contemporaries in glamorous locations. Maybe.

The fact remains, I *am* ambivalent. The uncomfortable truth is that my views on tweakments occupy the problematic space between distaste and envy. I'm like a Puritan who, in between convulsing with disapproval, longs for a bit of gold and velvet, and maybe some feasting. And so for the purposes of this book, or so I told myself – perhaps I'd been fishing about for an excuse all along – I thought I'd go and see what a practitioner I trust thought I should have done to my face. The reason I trust him is that he has done impeccable work to some faces I know intimately – the kind of work that makes you think, 'They look incredibly well,' way before you think, 'Hang on, I wonder if they've had something done.' Crucially, at least for me, this practitioner knows when to stop, and discourages his clients from having procedures he considers unnecessary.

This is not a given, and is important because having tweakments is completely addictive. Don't listen to anyone who tells you otherwise. After each one – well, allowing for downtime* – you think, 'Wow, that looks so much better. I should have done it years ago. I feel great. Now, what else shall I fix?' and unless you have someone saying, 'No, I'd leave it at that,' you can eventually end up looking mighty peculiar, as well as being seriously out of pocket. In theory the someone is a close friend but that doesn't always work, partly because it is actually quite

---

* This being the time spent at home watching Netflix in a darkened room after a cosmetic procedure while evidence of said procedure dies down. No downtime: back at work straight afterwards. Long downtime: several box sets.

difficult to say, 'I think you should take a break now,' without causing offence (because you're really saying, 'You're on the verge of looking super-weird,' which isn't something anyone wants to hear), and partly because if you see the person very regularly, you slightly stop seeing what they look like because you get used to the changes in their face too quickly.

So, a practitioner who is interested in your face looking its best and no further is an excellent ally. Again, such people are thin on the ground, since it involves them virtuously turning down lucrative work. So do ask any prospective practitioner what they would do if they had carte blanche, in order of priority, then tell them your budget and ask what they would do for that specific amount, and what difference it would make, and where. Beware also of the person who reels off a great giant list of everything that is 'wrong' with your face. There is nothing wrong with your face. The point of the exercise is to make you feel intrigued or excited by the possibilities provided by a few tweaks, not utterly depressed by the scale of the so-called 'problem' and the bottomless pit of money it would require to so-called 'correct' it. There should not be a hard sell. The idea isn't to make you feel shit. You want to feel like the person is looking forward to making you look your best, not like you're some catastrophe that they're duty-bound to try to tidy up as a kindness to society.

Injectables and me (Part Two)

Anyway, off I trotted to Harley Street 'for the *Beauty Edit*'. I'll be candid: in my head, I expected the doctor to let out a low whistle of admiration when I told him I was fifty-seven. I thought he might say, 'To be honest, I don't think you need anything done. Maybe a tiiiiny bit of Botox in that frown line – but really only so you haven't had a wasted train journey. I wouldn't consider it at all essential. Are you really fifty-seven?' Here he might shake his head, filled with awe, and call his assistant in: 'Look at this! This patient is pushing sixty. I know. Incredible.' And then they'd stare at me in wonderment.

What he actually said was that my skin was 'not too bad'. I had some obvious sun damage, here and here, oh, and also here and here (and here). There was age- and gravity-related loss of volume in my face, whose musculature had changed to accommodate it. My lateral eyelid – the beauty singular is like the fashion singular: a trouser, an eyelid – was drooping a bit as a result of the excessive strength that had developed at the side of my eyes, for example. My forehead had lost volume – yes, this is actually a thing – meaning it would be good to act now to prevent a 'peaked' appearance as a result of compensatory contraction of the forehead muscles 'to support heavy brows resulting from volume change and gravity'.

The thing that really surprised me, though, was that the long and deep line that went all the way from the inner corner of my eye diagonally down to halfway between the bottom of my nose and the bottom of my cheekbone was not, as I thought, some unfortunate fatness line but rather existed because of – you've guessed it – loss of volume. Put simply, loss of volume in some bits of the face makes other bits of the face develop super-strength to compensate, which makes things look slightly different. This happens around bony prominences, like your cheekbones and your jaw. Plus my orbital margin (around my eyes) had widened a little. Effectively your face kind of slides down a bit, and what that means is our friends the nose-to-mouth lines deepening, the arrival of a malar groove – the name for the line that wasn't in fact a mysterious fatness line – and the corners of the mouth downturning, giving one a peeved, disapproving expression in repose, like a cross dowager duchess.

To cut to the chase: I had Botox in my frown line, in the (small) lines at the sides of my eyes – specifically to prevent droopage, rather than because they were excessively crinkly – and in my forehead. The doses were small, meaning I can still frown and don't have one of those spooky, tight, shiny foreheads that semaphore: 'Hi, it's me, full of BOTOX. Yes, I've had BOTOX. Do you see? Right here! BOTOX, and plenty of it!' Then I had deep filler – you can hear it going in because the tissue carries the sound to your inner ear: tap tap tap tap POP – in my mid-face, near my cheekbones, to replace some of the lost volume that had led to the sodding malar groove, and a softer filler in the corners of my mouth. The doctor said that once all this had settled, we should look at a tiny bit of soft filler directly under the eye, near the tear trough, to fill out that particular hollow, and possibly at something called Morpheus8, which is a form of microneedling.*

My visible sun damage – a few freckle-sized brown dots on one side of my face and on my chin – *could* conceivably be helped by laser, he said but, as I would hope from anyone who knew their stuff, he didn't recommend it with my skin colour, as it could sometimes exacerbate the problem (see page 79). 'The thing is,' he said cheerily, 'that when it comes to tweakments it's quite easy to look dead if you have too much done. Your skin becomes too perfect, too undamaged, too smooth. Your face goes too tight. It's creepy.' We agreed to let my sun spots be, and I left liking them a lot better (brave protectors against death-skin!).

What do I think? I love it, goddammit. I think that the filler in that particular spot is a miracle. I hated that malar groove, but since I didn't know what a malar groove was, it never occurred to me that I could do anything about it. Having it filled has, to my eye, significantly improved how

---

* Microneedling is like it sounds: a roller that has needles on it piercing the skin and making thousands of tiny holes to maximize the efficacy of skincare or stimulate, as per, collagen production. Shorter needles for the first, longer for the second (you get slathered in numbing cream first). I can't say I fancy it, but I've seen the difference it can make: it does work. And, yes, it does hurt.

I look, in a way that you can't quite put your finger on – but if you know, which obviously I do, you can see very clearly that a whole unflattering deep groove has pretty much disappeared. My face hangs off my cheekbones better, for want of a more elegant explanation. The Botox is brilliant, with my frown softened and the skin around my eyes smoothed, but not creepily so. The corners of my mouth are horizontal, with no downward drag.

Will I go back when it all wears off? Yes, I think I will. I'm still not 100 per cent comfortable with the whole tweakment business, but it occurs to me that maybe part of acceptance is accepting that you're vain.*

TWEAKMENTS: USEFUL RESOURCES

I have only ever had Botox and filler. Everything in this book is tested on myself, so I don't feel qualified to comment at length on other procedures that are available – and there are a ton of them, with press releases about new

---

* If you've been wondering who I saw for several long paragraphs, it was Dr David Jack in London. I couldn't recommend him more highly. He says 80 per cent of his client base is women of a certain age who don't want their partners to know they have had anything done – men being grossly unobservant, the idea is that they look up from breakfast one morning and say, 'You're looking very well, darling. It must be that new dress.' That's pretty much all you need to know regarding the aesthetic he provides, other than he's a proper doctor, NHS-trained, who specialized in plastic and reconstructive surgery. His skincare line is pared-down (three basic products plus some extras) and highly effective.

See drdavidjack.com.

treatments pinging into my inbox more times per week than feels entirely sane. It is very easy to feel you 'have' to try this or that miracle-promising new procedure, which is a way of saying it's easy to end up permanently dissatisfied with the way you look and permanently chasing 'solutions' to 'problems' that either don't actually exist or are not realistically fixable. Obviously the newer a procedure, the less anyone knows about how it pans out several years down the line. So go easy. And remember this is an industry, one that, like the beauty industry, trades on women's insecurities – on the idea that you're not quite good enough as you are, and that if you only did this . . . and maybe this . . .

Having said all that:

- The absolute best way of finding someone good is via a personal recommendation. If you don't have anyone to ask, then:
- in the first instance always check your prospective practitioner's credentials with the Professional Standards Authority, professionalstandards.org.uk
- . . . and with the British College of Aesthetic Medicine, bcam.ac.uk
- saveface.co.uk list people who pass their 116-point assessment process
- There are also reviews on realself.com
- The beauty writer Alice Hart Davies is deeply knowledgeable in this area and has a useful, extremely detailed guide to tweakments and

recommended (by her) practitioners at
thetweakmentguide.com, featuring everything
from peels to thread lifts to fat-dissolving
injections

- If you are fascinated by this whole world and by
the minute detail of brand-new ingredients as well
as beauty more generally, I recommend subscribing
to Val Monroe's Substack, which is called How
Not To F*** Up Your Face. Monroe was for
sixteen years the beauty director of *O*, the Oprah
Winfrey magazine

There is no need whatsoever to have anything done
to your face if you don't want to. The people who love
you love your dear face exactly as it is, and if you sometimes catch a glimpse of yourself and think, 'Bloody
hell, what happened?' – well, literally every other woman
in the world has been there, or indeed *lives* there. It's fine.
It's ageing. It happens to every single living creature in
the universe. By all means have a little tweak if you fancy
it – if you don't like your involuntary frown, or your old
acne scars, or the texture of your skin, or whatever. Or
don't. That's fine too. It's *normal*.

PART 1
Skincare

CLEANSING

EXFOLIATION

SERUMS

MOISTURIZERS

OILY OR SPOT-PRONE SKIN

SUN DAMAGE AND SUN SPOTS

TWEAKMENTS

AT-HOME TREATMENTS

EYES

NECKS

Tweakments aside, there are now innumerable 'at home' treatments, many of them promising the sort of results that stop just short of booking in with a professional. Are any of them any good? Short answer: yes.

Let's start with masks, which have come a long, long way from the days when little sachets of clay-based masks were glued to the covers of teenage magazines. Nothing wrong with a clay-based mask, mind you. They're the business when it comes to drawing out impurities if you're very oily. In their more modern iterations, I rate **The Inkey List Kaolin Mask (around £5.50)** and **Beauty Pie's Super Pore Detox Purifying Black Clay Mask (around £13 to Beauty Pie members)**. Clay, being widely available, is cheap, hence these likeable prices. Serious ingredients unfortunately cost more.

I like masks that *do* stuff and am not very interested in masks that just feel quite nice if you've got ten minutes to kill in the bath before bed. If you're after one of those, I'd honestly just put on a thick layer of my favourite moisturizer and either tissue it off or, if there's not much excess once your bath has ended, go to bed with the leftovers still on.

THE EDIT: EIGHT EXCELLENT MASKS

- This product requires a klaxon, a banged gong and six people trumpeting a fanfare. The brand is **René Guinot**, which is only on my radar in the vaguest way in that some part of my brain is familiar with the packaging. Where from? Who knows? Maybe Brussels when I was younger. Maybe my stepmother used it. (She had very good skin, now I think of it, even though she fried it every summer on the beach.) Anyway, I haven't paid any attention to it ever, and clearly I have been missing a trick, because its **Masque Essentiel Nutri Confort (around £37)** is fricking amazing. It is brilliant to use if you're going out, but also brilliant if you're having one of those days or weeks when you look like crap for no reason that you can understand.

  It is a mask for knackered skin. You know the deal – grey, sallow, worn-out looking, and dry, so dry, looking like it desperately needs a holiday and some TLC. I tried it on my daughter's chronically dehydrated (due to indiscriminate DIY use of anti-spot products) skin – so thirsty that it had stopped feeling in any way elastic – and it performed a miracle in ten minutes. When she washed it off with a flannel, her skin was plump, boingy, luminous, and looked like it had just had a wholesome three-course meal. It was the kind of result I'd expect from a professional treatment, not sitting in the kitchen eating (unwholesome) crisps for ten minutes waiting for it to work. I did it again a week later, on the basis that you can't have enough plump, boingy luminosity, and the results were even better.

I was so delighted with this outcome that I tried the mask on myself, even though I don't have dry or knackered skin, to see what, if anything, would happen. And what happened was that I, too, had plumper, boingier, more luminous skin, to the point where it would be good never to be without a tube of this in the bathroom for (a) emergencies and (b) parties. Then – I'd got the bit between my teeth by this point – I thought I'd investigate Guinot's other masks, of which there are many. I went for **Masque Dynamisant Anti-Fatigue (around £49)**, which is a kind of instant pepper-up and works beautifully. I was raving to a friend about these important discoveries and she said she knew the brand well because she has a really red, reactive face and the only thing that works on it – and makes it not red – is the brand's **Crème Red Logic (around £67)**. I was amazed, never having thought of her as a person with a remotely red or reactive face, so there you go.

- **Natura Bissé Essential Shock Intense Mask (around £40).** This is another to keep on your bathroom shelf for emergencies – it's very good at revitalizing really dull, dreary, knackered skin.
- **Natura Bissé Diamond Instant Glow (around £80 for four treatments).** Near-miraculous. You get three little ampoules per go – one that contains a vigorous liquid exfoliator, one that hydrates and imparts (genuinely) instant radiance, and one that temporarily lifts the face, making it smooth and taut, or at least smoother and tauter. Really useful for big occasions. Natura Bissé, which is used in lots of spas, is a very good, slightly under-the-radar brand when it comes to at-home skincare. Serious results.
- **Beauty Pie Japanfusion™ 10 Minute Miracle Sheet Mask (around £7 for Beauty Pie members).** I don't love sheet masks because I rarely feel they provide the dramatic results I want if I'm going to sit there looking like an idiot, peering sadly out of what is basically a giant wet tissue with eyeholes. This one, though, is noticeably plumping and rehydrating (thanks to squalane and hyaluronic acid) and is a useful thing to have about your person if you've over-sunbathed, got a hangover, been on a long flight, or generally feel a bit desiccated. Makes your skin look plump

and milk-fed, like you should be twirling your plaits while wearing gingham and reclining on a hay bale.

- **Amanda Lacey Revealing Pink Mask (around £140).** Lacey is a top-notch facialist, who also makes a very good cleanser called **Cleansing Pomade (around £95).** This mask is full of fruit acids and also contains salicylic acid, both of which chomp away at dead skin cells. It isn't for the faint-hearted – it stings like billy-o – but I go back to it time and time again. The best way I can describe it is that it's like being slapped around the face – your skin tingles and then shakes itself wide awake, like a dog after swimming, before emerging at peak radiance.

- **Sarah Chapman Instant Miracle Mask (around £50 for a pack of four).** Chapman is another outstanding facialist. This mask, which was formulated for professional use, delivers on the promise of its title. It's got rhassoul in it, a kind of Moroccan clay (here called ghassoul) that is fantastic at everything – exfoliating, clarifying, tightening, deep cleaning – plus hyaluronic acid for moisture and magical vitamin C. You mix it up yourself. It is very good.

- **e.l.f. SuperMask with Centalla Asiatica (around £12).** This is for you if your face is red and uncomfortable – it is immediately calming and soothing.

- **Superdrug Vitamin E Leave-On Mask (about £3. You read that right)**. Serum-like mask that is packed with vitamin E, a multivitamin complex and horse-chestnut extract. Absolute bliss for dry or dehydrated skin.

Light therapy masks

These are those robot-looking light therapy masks that you charge, and which promise all sorts of impressive results. I haven't met one that does anything noticeable, but that's probably because I can't bring myself to test them properly, i.e. for a proper length of time. You're either the sort of person who is happy to watch telly peering out of the eyeholes of a piece of illuminated plastic glowing eerily on their face, or you're not. I'm not.

At-home face peels

A professional chemical face peel, courtesy of your friendly dermatologist, facialist or tweakment person, can be pretty hardcore. It involves removing part of the top layer of the skin through the use of acids, the idea being that collagen production is stimulated and new, fresh skin grows in its place. Professional peels vary in intensity – some use gentler acids than others – and in length of downtime. A lighter peel, which is still not something anyone should consider breezily, is good for helping large pores, fine lines and a degree of pigmentation; a deeper peel can be very effective at tightening skin up.

At-home peels need to be safe for a layperson to use, and are therefore necessarily weaker beasts than those designed to be administered by a licensed professional. That doesn't mean you can't still damage your skin, especially if you stupidly buy pro-grade kits from the internet. (I feel very confident that nobody reading this book would do this, but it's still worth saying.) Follow the instructions on the box to the letter, paying particular attention to what products you should stop using while you're peeling. Here are my favourites, though for what it's worth I'm slightly wary of at-home peels and rarely use them. Which isn't to say they aren't effective, because they are. Always be especially vigilant about sunscreen when you're using them – I would not use them in sunny weather. Your dead skin cells are being sloughed off and new skin is slowly being revealed underneath. That new skin is highly vulnerable to being damaged by the sun's rays, even if it's not a blazing-hot day. (Do remember – broken record, I know – that the sky doesn't have to be blue and glorious for rays to do their thing.)

THE EDIT: FIVE FANTASTIC PEELS

- **Dr Dennis Gross Alpha Beta Universal Daily Peel (around £20).** These are little pads infused with five different acids, both BHA and AHAs, as well as wrinkle-zapping ingredients like retinol. They are small but mighty, and despite their name I would use them two or three times a week rather than daily, and proceed with caution on very sensitive or reactive skin. They will help with pores and luminosity and you may see an improvement in fine lines. They would be my first entry-level choice.

- **Natura Bissé Glyco Extreme Peel (around £140).** This is a treatment – you use it twice a day for six weeks. Five different AHAs. Anti-ageing, smoothing, brightening. I would not use anything that says 'extreme' on sensitive skin. The clue's in the name: this is a Big Gun.

- **iS Clinical Active Peel System (around £85).** Two steps: first, deep exfoliation, then deep hydration. Contains copper tripeptide. Relatively gentle. This stuff is excellent on blackheads and poor texture.

- **Murad Resurgence Replenishing Multi-Acid Peel (around £50).** This feels oily, which I find comforting. Contains glycolic, malic and lactic acid for very effective results that leave skin feeling comfortable (not a given in this category).

- **The Ordinary AHA 30% + BHA 2% Peeling Solution (around £8.50).** This is a great, cheap, quasi-miraculous product that basically eats away all the gubbins clogging up your face and making your skin look dull.

AT-HOME HAIR REMOVAL

We'll keep it brief: this works. IPLs (intense pulsed light) came up in Sun Damage and Sun Spots (pages 69–81) but they can also be used anywhere you have unwanted hair, including on the face, as an alternative to professional laser hair removal. There are various IPL devices on the market, of which the best known is probably Phillips Lumea. The light from the device finds the pigment in the hair and zaps it, causing it to stop growing and fall out. You use the device once a fortnight for the first four treatments, and then touch up once every month or so. Obviously you need good lighting and to be quite meticulous. These devices are not, repeat not, suitable for darker skins, for the reasons outlined on page 79, though they can safely be used on olive and light brown skins. Always test on a tucked-away bit of underarm first, just in case.

PART 1

Skincare

CLEANSING

EXFOLIATION

SERUMS

MOISTURIZERS

OILY OR SPOT-PRONE SKIN

SUN DAMAGE AND SUN SPOTS

TWEAKMENTS

AT-HOME TREATMENTS

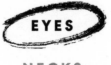 EYES

NECKS

Eyes and necks are two of the things that people ask about most often and, unhelpfully, two of the things that it's difficult to do anything seriously meaningful about once the neck or eye horse has bolted. What that means is that we can improve certain situations, but not reverse them using only cosmetics. Still, nothing wrong with an improvement.

I have never really believed in eye creams, as in dedicated creams for use around the eyes. The skin in this area is particularly delicate, like petals, and it has always seemed to me that all it needed every now and then – like, if I'd been out in the snow and wind – was the merest smidge of whatever moisturizer I was using on the rest of my face. If that. My basic principle has been 'It's too fragile – don't even touch it.' I have been told by more than one cosmetic practitioner that overuse of eye creams can lead to pouching and to fatty deposits under the eyes. But I've also been told quite authoritatively that using your normal moisturizer is a bad idea, like taking a sledgehammer to crack a nut, because the skin around your eyes is so much thinner and weedier than the skin on the rest of your face, and therefore needs a dedicated, much weedier cream.

So, if you have very dry skin around the eyes, by all means use a bog-standard separate eye cream, for the same reason that you use a moisturizer: we're trying to stop skin, wherever it is, from drying out and therefore developing (more) lines. Use it with a light hand, or rather a light middle finger, tapping extremely gently.

However: science evolves all the time, and there are now some very good eye creams and serums, mostly serums, containing specific active ingredients in quantities that are safe to use around the eye area. They are thinner and lighter than eye creams, therefore absorb much better, and usually address specific concerns.

THE EDIT: ONE FOR EVERYTHING

- **Estée Lauder Advanced Night Repair Eye Concentrate Matrix (around £60).** Highly effective on fine lines, whether they are crow's feet or under-eye wrinkles; great at helping with puffiness; good on dark circles too. The whole eye area looks tighter and more radiant. Clever, cooling applicator, too. A seriously good product.

THE EDIT: THREE FOR WRINKLES AND CRÊPINESS

- **Murad Retinol Youth Renewal Eye Serum (around £80).** Contains three different kinds of retinol/retinoids but is safe for sensitive skin. When I tested this it made a visible difference, much to my amazement, after about a month of use. Nothing earth-shattering, but there was a definite softening of my crow's feet, although I don't know how significant that is because my crow's feet weren't terribly deep in the first place. General tightening up too.

- **Medik8 Crystal Retinal® Ceramide Eye Serum (around £40, various strengths, start with the weakest, which isn't that weak).** This made a visible difference to my eye lines and to the texture of the area under my eyes.
- **No7 Pure Retinol Eye Cream (around £25).** This has retinol (0.5%) and collagen peptide. A good and well-priced all-rounder.

THE EDIT: FOUR FOR DARK CIRCLES

Remember the magical brightening powers of vitamin C (turn to page 40 if you need a reminder)? It follows that it can – and does – help with dark circles, though there isn't anything that will obliterate them permanently (although a good concealer can work like PhotoShop. See page 39). Try:

- **Medik8 C-Tetra® Eye Serum (around £20).** Yes, Medik8 again. It's an excellent brand and this is an excellent eye serum.
- **Ole Henriksen Banana Bright™ + Eye Crème (around £35).** A cream, not a serum, but it contains three types of vitamin C, plus . . . real gold. Yes.

Gold is supposed to aid vitamin C delivery but is also, being gold, pleasingly and efficiently luminizing. It works on everyone, but I massively rate the whole Banana Bright range on darker skins.

- **Garnier Brightening 4% Vitamin C, Niacinamide, Caffeine and Banana Powder Eye Cream (around £10).** This one is very good at de-puffing as well as brightening.
- **Paula's Choice C5 Super Boost Eye Cream (around £40).** An excellent all-rounder that makes you look rested.

There are many more, at all sorts of prices, but you get the idea: vitamin C is a good friend to dark circles.

THE EDIT: ONE FOR EMERGENCIES:

- **Erborian Ginseng Eye Patch (around £6.50).** Temporarily smoothes and de-puffs in about fifteen minutes. See also **Peter Thomas Roth**, page 120.

For dark circles if you have Asian or Black skin

Obviously all of the skincare products I am recommending work on darker skins – I test them on myself, and I have brown skin. However, dark circles involve concealer, and not all concealer is created equal when it comes to melanin levels. Black and brown people often have thinner skin on their bottom eyelids and are predisposed to hyper-pigmentation in this specific area – it's called periorbital hyper-pigmentation and is related to having higher levels of melanin (skin pigment). The circles/shadows sometimes have a greyish tinge. However, as someone half Pakistani, I am not 100 per cent convinced that anyone should feel embarrassed about the dark shadows under their eyes, or even try to conceal them. There is no longer a rule that says everyone has to conform to Western beauty standards or else, for which I give daily thanks to all the people working so hard to celebrate inclusivity and diversity. I say that as someone who couldn't buy foundation to match my skin tone until I was in my mid-twenties, and even then initially only in the US, and who used to compare my chunky Asian earlobes to the non-existent earlobes of my school friends and feel ashamed of them. Bollocks to that, and bollocks to feeling like dark shadows must at all costs be heavily concealed. If you *do* want to conceal them, though – also fine! it's all fine! – then picking even a fractionally wrong shade can exacerbate the greyness or ashiness. There is a comprehensive guide to concealers on page 153.

For puffiness and/or bagginess

This is going to sound obvious, but do check that you're not allergic to either your pillow or to skincare or makeup that you're using regularly, because that is absolutely a thing that happens and that is more common than you'd think (as is not drinking enough water and/or eating too much salt, but I'm not your mum).

The thing to know about eye bags is that there are two sorts: one that you can't do anything about without a trip to a cosmetic surgeon, and one that you sort of can. Type 1 is to do with the structure of your face changing with age. The eye orbit lives in something called the orbital septum, which provides the architecture for the whole area, including the fat pads everyone has under their eyes. The orbital septum gets weaker as we age, which can have the effect of pushing the fat pads forwards and into a more prominent position. These are the really stubborn, quite solid-feeling, half-moon-shaped under-eye bags that it is pointless to try to address through skincare. They are a physical lump, and if yours are very bad or bother you greatly, the solution is a lower blepharoplasty, which is plastic surgery to remove them. Everything I said about finding a good tweakment provider applies in triplicate to plastic surgeons. Your first port of call is BAAPS, the British Association of Aesthetic Plastic Surgeons, baaps.org.uk.

The second type of eye bags relates to lack of sleep, stress, screen time, pollution – you know the drill – and sometimes to water retention (especially if you wake up puffy and are de-puffed by teatime. Sleeping with your head raised higher can help). In any case, what happens is that the blood vessels under the eye dilate, which means the area swells and can become inflamed. As with any swelling, you need to cool it down in the hope that the vessels will contract again, thus causing the puffiness to abate. The two best ways of achieving this in the under-eye area are with coldness and products containing caffeine, which makes things shrink. (The quest for shrink-age is also why that trope about using haemorrhoid cream on your eye bags exists. Maybe a makeup artist once did this on a shoot in an emergency situation and everyone got very excited, but please don't do it at home.) We may think of cold teabags, cold cucumber slices and cold com-presses as comically old-fashioned, but they all work (up to a point) in the short term. Caffeine is faster. A combin-ation of the two is ideal. Keep these products in the fridge to maximize their cooling powers.

THE EDIT: FOUR EYE LIFE-SAVERS

- **The Inkey List Caffeine Eye Serum (around £10)** and **The Ordinary Caffeine 5% + EGCG (around £7.90)**. Both of these do the job well before a big event or night out.
- **Dr Dennis Gross Hyaluronic Marine Dew It All Eye Gel (around £60)**. Very good, though at a price. Results last up to seventy-two hours. Hyaluronic acid, as I've said before, attracts water to skin; caffeine de-puffs; Japanese algae helps with suppleness. Contains optical diffusers to help with luminosity.

- **L'Oréal Revitalift Filler Eye Serum 2.5% [Hyaluronic Acid and Caffeine] (around £25).** This is the world's bestselling eye serum. Pleasant-to-use applicator that looks slightly like anal beads. Sits nicely under makeup.
- **Peter Thomas Roth Instant FirmX Eye (around £32).** This one periodically goes viral. You put a tiny bit of the gel on and your under-eye is temporarily tightened and firmed, rather as if you'd used face tape or liquid glue. You mustn't move your face an inch while it dries, and be extremely light-handed applying makeup to the area once it has dried. Not especially comfortable – it feels a bit like dry egg white – but it absolutely works and will last all evening.

PART 1
Skincare

CLEANSING

EXFOLIATION

SERUMS

MOISTURIZERS

OILY OR SPOT-PRONE SKIN

SUN DAMAGE AND SUN SPOTS

TWEAKMENTS

AT-HOME TREATMENTS

EYES

NECKS

Ah, necks. I bow to no one in my admiration of Nora Ephron, but rereading *I Feel Bad About My Neck*, a collection of essays about ageing published in 2006, when she was sixty-five, is quite sobering. I remember the book as a brutally candid, deeply hilarious masterpiece, which it remains – but, wow, Ephron (1941–2012) is hard on herself and on womankind generally. Attitudes that seemed perfectly normal in 2006 now feel wildly dated, and a little bit sad. Ephron says, for instance, that you're okay wearing a bikini until you're thirty-four, at which point you have nine more years to show off before the need to cover up becomes imperative. Necks must be hidden from the age of forty-three ('Our faces are lies and our necks tell the truth'), and that is that: nothing more to be done except wear polo-necks. At the end of the essay called 'On Maintenance' ('Maintenance is what you have to do just so you can walk out the door knowing that if you go to the market and bump into a guy who once rejected you, you won't have to hide behind a stack of canned food'), Ephron passes a homeless woman in the street. The woman has grey hair, a moustache, bushy eyebrows, dirty nails, a pot belly. 'I am exactly eight hours away from looking like that woman on the street,' Ephron notes, having already listed the effort and vast expense she goes to in order to, as she sees it, remain presentable. Obviously much and perhaps even most of this is for comic effect, but revisiting the book, I was really struck by the depth of Ephron's anxieties. She was sixty-five and had a marvellous life. Why the self-disgust, the compulsion to hide 'imperfect' body parts, the need to compare herself to someone homeless and desperate? I really hope that the number of people who still think like this is dwindling. Being in a state of near-panic about ageing is not a good use of one's time. The stress of it probably ages you faster, too.

Having said all that, necks *are* challenging. One minute they're just a neck, usefully holding up your head, going about their business discreetly. The next their texture has changed into crêpe de Chine. There might be a little bit of wattle action, too. This seems to happen overnight, while you weren't paying proper attention. Now what? Is it too late? Is there anything you can do about it, short of having a neck lift? The absolutely blunt truth is that, if you want to make a clear and visible difference to your neck, your best ally might be a type of filler called Profilho, which is like injecting serious moisture, with the plumping and firming effects that suggests. I've not had it, so that's all I'm able to say about it. I am resistant to the idea of needles in the neck, even though

I'm okay with them in the face,* but I have a friend who swears by Profilho and whose neck bears testament to its impressive powers.

I find it helps to remember that no one likes their neck. The actor and model Isabella Rossellini was sacked as the face of Lancôme for being too old at forty-three, and rehired when she was sixty-three and Lancôme had just got a new CEO (a woman, obviously, for the first time in the company's history). Rossellini gave an interview in 2022, when she was seventy, in which she talked about ageing. Many women's dream, she said, was to 'be young – not to grow old', but Isabella preferred the dream of 'grow[ing] old with beauty and dignity and elegance'. She said she was ageing naturally and hadn't even had Botox because it would be hypocritical, given that she lives on an organic farm. 'We all age. It's part of nature,' she said. 'I've never done any plastic surgery. If you do it, you might win a battle, but you lose the war.'

All well and good. Except for necks. 'I have to confess, my neck is the thing that makes me sometimes think I should have plastic surgery,' she said. 'The neck is always a little bit upsetting, but I live with it. I prefer a little scarf to an operation.'

* 'Do I contradict myself?/Very well then I contradict myself,/(I am large, I contain multitudes).' From Walt Whitman's 'Song of Myself', 51. Useful in arguments as well as in discussions about injectables.

Neck Creams

I never really paid much attention to my neck. I've always just taken my normal moisturizer down to my collarbone or thereabouts (when I remembered to, so maybe twice a month, if we're honest) and hoped for the best. And now, to paraphrase Nora, I feel bad about it. Now, ageing is ageing and I don't want to care that much about two centimetres of potentially wattly neck, any more than I want to care about wrinkles around my eyes or laughter lines. You need to be able to differentiate between things that you dislike and that are fixable – huge frown lines that make you look grumpy, maybe, or the dreaded marionette lines (see page 89) – and things that, in the great scheme of things, either don't really matter, like eye wrinkles – I mean, so what, really? – or are actively nice, like evidence that you've spent a good part of your life laughing.

But necks sag. While that's not as annoying as looking permanently furious or suddenly developing Victorian-looking jowls, it's not as nice as the friendlier wrinkles and lines.

Necks really need attention from the age of about thirty onwards – tell your daughters to use a neck cream, or just to run their moisturizer down to their collarbone as a matter of course (and not taking the bi-monthly option favoured by my younger self). There are fewer oil glands on necks than on faces, meaning they lose elasticity faster, plus they really don't like UV rays, for which reason you should also take your sunscreen to your collarbone rather than just concentrate it on your face. It won't make things better – too late, I'm afraid – but at least it won't make them worse.

If your neck is not something you've previously paid attention to, you can somewhat improve its texture and firmness but, alas, there isn't a product that smoothes and tightens it back to its former glory.

Quite special: one product to give us hope

Murad Retinal ReSculpt™ Overnight Treatment (around £105). I'm quite excited by this product from one of my most trusted brands. It has been developed especially for 'advanced' signs of ageing, and is neck-specific, though it also visibly smoothes wrinkles and crêpy skin on the face. The neck 'n' jowl results, though, are seriously impressive. I tested this for four weeks and saw, with my own eyes, a noticeable lifting and tightening effect. It has made me rethink what might be possible in terms of hoicking and firming this most traditionally un-hoickable, stubbornly un-firmable area.

THE EDIT: FOUR EXCELLENT NECK CREAMS

- **Prai's Ageless Throat & Decolletage Crème (around £25).** When I reviewed this for my Style column, I used it for just over two weeks, but religiously and twice a day. There are many permutations of this cream, including a heavier night version, one with retinol, and also a more serum-like concentrate, but I was using the day one. Prai is an excellent brand generally, fairly priced and results-based, and this particular cream has won several awards. And – to my surprise, I must say – it did seem to make a perceptible difference.

Now, before you go rushing out to score a miracle in a jar, 'perceptible' doesn't mean 'dramatic' or 'I now have the neck of a teenager.' What it means is that my neck looked, to my eye, less knackered and a little bit firmer. The potentially wattly bit still looked potentially wattly – as I said, I expect that in order to swerve wattliness altogether I should have paid attention to my neck twenty years ago. But! The *texture* improved and the whole neck arrangement looked as if it had had a nourishing drink that somehow made it stand up straighter. It did not look the same as it does after I've applied normal moisturizer to it. It was definitely tauter – a *little* tauter (I really don't want to oversell this product). You need only a tiny bit, and with its reasonable price tag, I'd say it's good insurance for the future.

- I also highly rate **StriVectin TI Advanced Tightening Neck Cream Plus (around £80)**, which does somewhat fade the appearance of those horizontal lines that are a bit like the rings in a tree, and also has some effect on neck sag. You should see an improvement, but not a miracle.

- Also impressive: **Beauty Pie Über Youth™ Neck and Chest Super Lift Serum Spray (around £17.50 to Beauty Pie members)**, which contains every neck-improving ingredient known to mankind, is made in Switzerland by special neck boffins (maybe) and does seem to have tightening and lifting powers. It is also good at targeting sun damage on the chest, though as I was saying earlier, the upper chest is hard to fix entirely.
- **Neostrata Skin Active Triple Firming Neck Cream (around £50)** has such fanatical devotees that I feel I should mention it even though I haven't used it myself.

It may sound obvious, but the best way to distract from a neck you dislike is to give people other focal points: jewellery and scarves, maybe some statement earrings. Or, most obviously, your lovely face. At the end of the day, it's only a neck. There's no need to feel that bad about it.

PART 2

Makeup

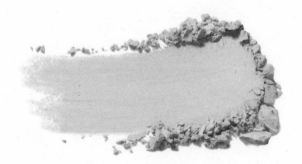

If skincare is structural engineering – making sure your house is solid and isn't going to fall down any time soon – then makeup is the fun part: decorating. As with decorating, it is easy to completely change the appearance of a room/face with minimal effort, but unlike with decorating, you're never stuck with one look. You can go from minimalist to showgirl in half an hour. Makeup is just so *fun*.

Most people our age *are* stuck with one look, though. We do the makeup equivalent of really wanting a new sofa but not being quite sure what the sofa should be like, or where to get it from, or in what colour, and so we sit looking at the old sofa and thinking, 'Ah, well, it does its job, I suppose. It's not actively horrible. And it *is* comfy. Let's just stick with it.'

There is just so much damn makeup around – look for a new eye pencil online and you will be presented with hundreds, if not thousands, of choices. How would you even go about picking one? Stand-alone beauty shops are a bit better – at least there are humans on hand to ask, and at least you can touch and feel the products – but they can also be intimidating. People worry about being encouraged to buy items they don't really need at prices they can't really afford, or that they'll leave with six things when they only went in for one. Also, you feel stupid standing in a shop and asking the charming twenty-three-year-old assistant, 'What actually *is* contour?' or whatever, sounding like your grandma to your own ears.

It's frustrating. How hard can it be to find a perfect foundation for your particular skin? You keep reading about advances in technology, in new textures and finishes, in massively expanded shade ranges, but nothing you try seems to quite work for you – too thick, too watery, too much coverage, not enough. Too shiny, too matte, too creepily long-lasting, disappears by lunchtime. And so on, applied to every single product you might want to put on your face.

Then you get to the *how* you put it on your face, which is half the battle. Beauty influencers do excellent work explaining, in detail and on camera, how to go about achieving a particular look. These little films have an almost hypnotic quality, and they are undoubtedly full of helpful tricks and tips. But (a) the person by definition really knows what they're doing, which isn't necessarily the case with you, the inexpert person watching at home; (b) you feel a bit too old to be sitting there in the bathroom trying to copy some younger person doing their makeup – you've got things to be getting on with, it's not like you care that much, you just want to look nice; and (c) you can't help noticing that they wear an awful lot of makeup. I mean, my God. So. Much. Makeup.

I always think, 'They look amazing, but that's about twenty-five different products, and I don't have the time, the inclination or, more to the point, the need to look that polished and "done" every day.' I think it's important to wear the makeup that fits your life, not the makeup you'd wear in some imaginary version of it (this also applies to clothes and interiors, in my view). And so, (d), you end up thinking, 'It should be easier than this. I'm an adult woman who's worn makeup for decades. I shouldn't be watching videos on my phone, and I don't care about the latest viral product. I just want my face to look a bit better. Why is it so hard?'

At this point, a degree of exasperation sets in and you decide to, as it were, stick with the old sofa. Sounds familiar? Stand by. We're going to break it down.

But, first, I should point out that there is a difference, I think, between 'performing' beauty, which is a bit like drag, and just looking like a good version of yourself. I'm less interested in the former because, fun as it is sometimes, it's too much for most people's everyday life. Most of us don't need to draw on features we don't have, or to wear false lashes as a matter of course – though we will go into both of these, because there may be times when knowing how to put them on comes in mighty handy. So in the pages that follow, my focus will be more on *being* and less on performing, though with some exceptions.

Right. Let's get into it. Before we start, I have just one observation: the older you get, the less makeup you need. This is because makeup makes you look older, as we all remember from being fourteen. You need very good makeup, judiciously applied – but less of it. Happily for us, that makes things a lot easier.

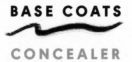

Great skin is everything

Do I need something under my foundation? Obviously this all depends on what you're going to spend your day doing. If you're going to be sitting in the garden with your book, all you need is sunscreen and a big hat. But otherwise, I say yes. It really helps. As you will have gathered, I am obsessed with good skin, including creating the illusion of good skin where no good skin is available, to the point where I deeply believe that good skin is what really makes good makeup. It's the largest piece of real estate on your face, so it follows that if your skin looks amazing, you're going to feel great. Also, there is nothing more ageing than skin that looks tired or thirsty. And full faces of heavy-duty makeup not only look very dated and uncool but are tremendously ageing. It's really worth focusing on everything that makes optimal perky, fresh skin more likely, and for me that very much includes pre-foundation products, mostly but not exclusively primers. The other thing about primer is that if you've gone to the trouble and expense of using the best skincare you can afford, primer seals it in.

THE EDIT: EIGHT
FAVOURITE PRIMERS

- **Elemis Superfood Glow Priming Moisturizer (around £40).** I am particularly into this ultra-light, brightening moisturizer/primer, which feels lovely on the skin. You can use it as a moisturizer, i.e. all over your face, or you can use it as a primer, under everything, or you can use it strategically to impart a bit of wholesome glow to selected areas of your face, so more like a highlighter. I find dedicated highlighters (see page 209) are often alarming unless you really know what you're doing – it's quite easy to look laminated and/or slightly futuristic, which isn't necessarily what you want when you've only nipped out to buy some milk. No such worries here: this is an entirely manageable, hard-to-mess-up amount of flattering, nicely lit emphasis, even if you just slap it on all over without paying much attention and don't use anything else on top. Note: Elemis say to apply the product in upward strokes.

  I use it under makeup, and I love it because it makes my skin look awake and well rested. The level of dewiness (see page 143) it imparts is just right. You'll look golden and glowy in an entirely appropriate way.

- **Charlotte's Magic Serum Crystal Elixir by Charlotte Tilbury (around £30).** If it's a serum, what's it doing here? The answer is that it's a serum designed to go under makeup. It is a relative of the same brand's **Charlotte's Magic Cream**, which many people love but which I find too rich in its original version (it now comes in an oil-free one). This serum contains vitamin C, niacinamide and various other hydrating, illuminating ingredients, as well as a 'crystal complex' of various minerals that impart just the right amount of luminosity.

- **Hollywood Flawless Filter by Charlotte Tilbury (around £40).** This has been a cult product pretty much since the day it launched back in 2018. It has recently been reformulated (still works like a dream, which is just as well as otherwise there would be riots). It's a foundation-primer-highlighter mash-up that is hard to describe but that very cleverly makes you look slightly airbrushed while at the same time just giving you lovely skin. You can wear it on its own, under foundation or on top of it, and you can put it on all over or just wherever you want to blur imperfections or impart radiance. Amazing on cheekbones. Amazing full stop, actually – this is one of the few products I wouldn't be without. Like being followed about by your own personal lighting crew.

- **e.l.f. Halo Glow Liquid Filter (around £14)** is *veeeery* similar to the **Hollywood Flawless Filter**. At this price you really can't go wrong. Wide shade range.
- **Hourglass Mineral Veil Primer (around £23)**. This is an excellent primer. It is light, oil-free, glides on like a dream and does its job beautifully – fills in small lines, creates a smooth surface for makeup to adhere to, helps conceal pores, tones down redness, provides a perfect base. It also turns your makeup waterproof because it's water-repellent, which I call clever. See also **Hourglass Vanish Airbrush Primer (around £23)** which is particularly good at controlling shine and at smoothing unevenly textured skin – you can really see the difference when you put makeup on top.
- **Erborian CC Red Correct (around £20)**. Erborian is a brilliant Korean-French beauty brand (see page 145) and one of my favourites. This colour-correcting cream is a marvel under makeup on reddened fair skin, including rosacea, though it is less good if your skin is dark. But if you're white-skinned and always have what used to be called 'high colour' (see page 144), meet your new best friend.
- **Beauty Pie Wonderfilter™ Velvet Finish Primer (around £12.50 to Beauty Pie members)**. This stuff is particularly good at

blurring large pores. I know everyone thinks they have massive pores even when their pores are perfectly normal-sized, but if you really do have large pores, this is for you. Completely matte. Like Polyfilla, basically, including on fine lines.

- **Laura Mercier Pure Canvas Primer (around £30).** There are five of these, each addressing a different concern – Hydrating, Illuminating, Blurring, Perfecting and Protecting (SPF50). They are all excellent.
- **Ole Henriksen Banana Bright Face Primer (around £31).** This illuminating, vitamin C-packed primer is particularly good on brown skin, for reasons I can't specifically explain. You'll just have to take my word for it. Good on other skins too, obviously, but if you happen to have darker skin and to be casting about for a new primer, do give it a try. I think you'll be pleased. The whole Banana Bright range is outstanding, as I was saying on page 116. I love this primer.

'DEWY' SKIN

Dewy skin has become *de rigueur*, though at the time of writing there does seem to be a small breakaway sect that is heading back towards matte. We'll get to my views on matteness and older skin a bit later on. I am in favour of dewiness. But I've tried out so many products over the last couple of years that impart such crazy amounts of dewiness that your skin literally looks wet (that's the polite description) or insanely greasy and sweaty (the realistic one). With these products, if you look in the mirror and ask yourself, 'I know it's a look, but I wonder, do I look a bit sweaty?' then knock them on the head because, yes, chances are that you do. If it's occurred to you, it will occur to other people.

There is so much written about, and so many products are designed to produce, dewy, radiant, glassy, etc., etc., skin, but the truth is that many of these make the average middle-aged woman look downright odd. This is because you have to be really careful with simulated dewiness once your skin is no longer dewy on its own. It has to look ultra realistic. This is often a problem with older skin, or indeed with older hair or older clothing. You can't just go, 'I want the skin/hair/clothes I had when I was twenty,' and assume that your wish will magically come true. You more usually just end up looking a bit weird.

What works for a red face

A red face is what ladies of a certain generation used to call 'high colour' and is the bane of some people's lives. Stuccoing your face with serious concealer and high-coverage foundation is one solution, but this is a particular look and requires a hefty and sure-footed application of other makeup, since you can't walk around with only heavy-duty foundation on. It makes your features disappear and you have to draw them back in, which is great if you're a drag artist but not ideal at 8 a.m. when you're going about your ordinary day.

Anyway: what I'd do if I had a red face is colour-correct. Erborian's green colour corrector, **Erborian Red Correct (about £20)**, is a good option under foundation. **Cicapair Tiger Grass Colour Correcting Treatment by Dr Jart+ (around £17)** is a beefier one. This is also green. (Colour wheel, innit? If you were accidentally orange, you'd tone it down with blue, which should have been a thing in the early 2000s.) It comes in a tub rather than a tube. Like Erborian, Dr Jart+ is an excellent Korean skincare brand. The anti-redness products contain a trademarked Green Re.pair Solution, which is a mix of Tiger Grass, various herbs and minerals, a humectant and a probiotic. This cream does that weird thing of completely changing your skin tone, so that redness and irritation are dramatically reduced and replaced by smooth, even skin. The effect isn't purely aesthetic – the cream is a treatment rather than a primer or moisturizer, though it works as both of those too. You can wear foundation on top, but it won't need to be heavy and you may not need it at all.

If you don't have a red face, by the way, or only a very slightly red one or one that's red in odd patches, this also works as a smoothing, evening-out preparation, and the above remark applies – you may find you don't need anything on top. If your face is mega-red, there's a whole Cicapair range, including an excellent serum.

Eye primer

First, do you need it? Assuming you wear eye makeup, the answer is yes if your eyelids have 'texture', i.e. are crinkly. There's nothing wrong with a crinkly eyelid, but it does not provide a smooth base for any eye makeup you may want to apply to it. Said makeup will not glide on, which will both annoy you and emphasize the creases. Also yes if your eye makeup doesn't stay put. And primer helps enormously if your eyelids are in any way discoloured. Most people's are – there are darker and lighter bits, and primer provides a smooth, clear, uniform surface for makeup to glide onto and stick to, kind of like a base coat before you go in with the proper paint colour. Eye primer is really worth buying – the difference it makes is notable. Also, if you're wearing an exciting eyeshadow or liner, it will show it off to its best effect. (It will also stop anything remotely glittery from dropping.) And, no, it isn't just normal primer in a smaller tube: face primers are all about slip; eye primers are all about grip.

THE EDIT: FOUR OF THE BEST EYE PRIMERS

- **NARS Smudge Proof Eyeshadow Base (around £23).** Seriously good.
- **Urban Decay Eyeshadow Primer Potion (around £19).** One from the vaults, and none the worse for that. I know people who refuse to use anything else.
- **Milani Eyeshadow Primer (around £10).** A decent cheaper alternative.
- **NYX Professional Makeup Eyeshadow Base (around £5).** Pretty good for a fiver.

Makeup

BASE COATS

CONCEALER

TINTED MOISTURIZERS AND SKIN TINTS

FOUNDATIONS

BRONZERS

BLUSH

HIGHLIGHTERS, LUMINIZERS AND
CONTOUR

BROWS

EYELASHES

EYELINERS

EYESHADOWS

LIPS

FAKE TAN

You may not need foundation at all!

Why do we wear foundation? Because we want great skin, and we feel insecure, perhaps especially so as we age, about the greatness of our own. Foundation gives the illusion of a lovely, smooth, even expanse, with nary an imperfection to spoil the view. And that is great – if the foundation is good and applied correctly rather than sitting in one's creases making everything worse, which we'll get to in a bit (and which is why primer is helpful). But I want to run an idea past you first.

What we think of as great skin – peachy, luminous, poreless – is the skin belonging to every young person. On an older person, someone in middle age or beyond, that kind of skin does not look great. It looks strange. I refer you back to my aesthetic doctor saying that too many tweakments could end up with skin so eerily taut and smooth that it looks dead. I think the same can be said of skin that is overly concealed and corrected with makeup. It develops an unearthly quality, like the skin that might be created to clothe an AI robot. You stop and stare, but not always in a good way.

I recently met a woman who must have been in her

eighties and who had extraordinary skin, completely unlined, like china or glass, not because she was a genetic anomaly but because she was rich and clearly spent a lot of time and money trying to buy back her youth, which she was very open about. The effect was unsettling: you think, 'Wow, great skin,' and then, 'for a twenty-two-year-old'. But the person is not twenty-two. They have an older person's hands, an older person's stance, rheumier eyes, thinner lips, a stoop . . . And then this extraordinary skin. It's too much. And I don't think you need to be in your eighties for it to be too much. There is such a thing as part of you looking too young, way younger than the rest of you, and it's jarring. On the face, you want to see life, not some vast expanse of improbable creaminess, like a lake of milk.

Concealer is built to conceal. It will cover anything you want covered, from darkness and shadows to blemishes, broken capillaries, redness, discoloured areas, brown spots, old scars and anything else you don't love the look of. It will do this better than foundation, since it is what it was invented to do. It is a mono-tasker, with one job and one job only. The textures of concealer are denser, they contain way more pigments, and the good ones don't budge. And, if you get a perfect match in terms of skin shade, it is entirely possible to bypass foundation altogether: the bits you want to conceal are concealed, and all that's left is lovely natural skin.

When I am at home just going about my ordinary day, I usually wear only concealer. I might add the Erborian

BB cream on page 160 if I have social events to go to, but generally I find that not having foundation on my skin makes it look younger and more alive.

Now, obviously, this concealer-only business is easier said than done: your concealer needs to be exceptional if it's all you're going to use, so you need to put some effort into finding The One. Colour aside, you should pick something that works perfectly on your skin, so your skin type is relevant here: something too rich will slide off oilier skin, just as something too dry will only accentuate dehydration. Remember that some concealers are for concealing, and others are for brightening. The shortlist below should cover all eventualities. Please note, some of these are too heavy or dense to use on the delicate skin under your eyes – I've marked which ones are and aren't suitable, and there are dedicated eye concealers on page 157. These are the ones I like to use when I'm not using anything else. They are also perfect if you want to use something sheer on the rest of your face, meaning you can use much lighter and more flattering formulations if you're going to be wearing foundation. **Please note that all concealers, wherever you apply them, need to be set with loose powder to maximize longevity (see page 156 for my recommendation).**

THE EDIT: FIVE OF THE BEST CONCEALERS

- **Laura Mercier Flawless Fusion Ultra Longwear Concealer (around £30).** I swear by this for everyday use. Medium coverage. Comes in a tube with a nice doe-foot applicator. Light texture belies its covering powers, which last all day. I press this in with my finger, then tap it in with a damp sponge. Suits all skins, though maybe not super-oily. Good on under-eyes too.

- **Laura Mercier Secret Camouflage (around £32).** This has been around for ever and remains a total champ; I live in fear of them discontinuing it. Full coverage, very dense and heavily pigmented. This will hide anything and keep it hidden: I use it on my dark brown sun spots and they vanish. Despite its density, it does not sit awkwardly on the skin, though you do need to blend it in well. Comes in a dual palette – you mix the two colours until you reach the perfect match, then apply with a teeny-tiny brush. This is a minuscule faff, but it does mean you get the best possible shade match. Oil free. Suits all skins. The darkest shade is good but nowhere near dark enough for very Black skin. Way too much for under-eyes, in my view.
- **NARS Soft Matte Complete Concealer (around £26).** NARS are brilliant at concealers – the **Radiant Creamy Concealer (around £26)** is wonderful for under the eyes. But for me this is the heavy-duty hero, the one

that, much like **Secret Camouflage**, will make spots, scars, redness and dark marks disappear. Comes in twenty-six inclusive shades and contains peptides and hyaluronic acid. If you can't find a perfect match – unlikely but possible – it is worth going to the expense of buying two little pots and mixing them until you create the exact right shade, because concealer only works if it's exactly the same colour as your skin (this doesn't apply to the under-eye area, which can go a shade lighter). Suits all skins. Good on under-eyes used with the lightest hand, though I would favour **Radiant Creamy**, as above.

- **Kevyn Aucoin The Sensual Skin Enhancer (around £35).** Not a concealer as such, but the late makeup artist Kevyn Aucoin's little pot of luminescent, heavily pigmented cream – you need very, very little – works brilliantly as a sort of liquid skin Band-Aid on problem areas, provided your skin isn't super-oily and that the problems aren't glaring – it wouldn't be much use on a crater-like spot, for instance, but it would work perfectly on a discoloured patch. Dewy finish, very pretty, can also be mixed with moisturizer and applied all over for a wholesome glow, or used as highlighter if you buy one shade lighter than your skin tone. It's lovely on brow bones. Waterproof. This is good on lightly shadowed under-eyes because it's so skin-like, though bear in mind that it does have glow. It's quite thick and you really do need only a minuscule amount. Inclusive shade range. (It's really beautiful on Black skin.)

- **RMS UnCoverup Concealer (around £30).** This is a three-in-one concealer, tinted moisturizer and colour corrector that has a very skin-like finish and offers sheer to medium coverage. Excellent on shadows under the eyes, but also elsewhere on the face. Inclusive range of particularly well-thought-out colours. I like this clean beauty brand enormously, and its founder and creative director, Rose-Marie Swift, is inspirational – talk about ageing well. Now in her late sixties, she was a makeup artist for thirty years before founding the brand. She looks awesome, chic and polished but in a very natural way – do look her up.

Here are some more good concealers that work on under-eyes, bearing in mind that the bigger the shadows, the lighter the hand. Remember to set your concealer with a very little bit of powder – I have found **Laura Mercier's Translucent Loose Powder (around £34 for a giant pot)** unbeatable for well over a decade, which is why there are no other setting powders in this book – pressing it in with a tiny triangular powder puff of the kind you can buy cheaply on Amazon in packs of six.

THE EDIT: SEVEN OF THE BEST UNDER-EYE CONCEALERS

- **Maybelline Instant Age Rewind Eraser (around £9)**. Developed for older skins, hydrating and creamy, good coverage (but more darker shades, please).
- **IT Cosmetics Bye Bye Undereye Full Coverage Anti Ageing Waterproof Concealer (around £20)**. This is seriously heavy duty – too heavy duty for most people, I think. But if there's some sort of major under-eye catastrophe, this will certainly conceal it. It's really thick – you need to use a microscopic amount and blend like crazy to avoid it sitting there looking obvious. I would go over with a sponge afterwards (see page 160). Particularly good shade range at the darker end.
- **Hourglass Vanish Airbrush Concealer (around £34)**. By contrast, this stuff feels weightless. Extremely comfortable on the under-eye skin; crease-resistant and light-reflecting. Clever applicator. Inclusive shade range
- **Trinny London BFF Eye (around £28)**. This is an excellent serum-concealer hybrid – firming, hydrating, cooling – whose lovely light texture belies its heroic concealing powers. Twelve shades. Very skin-like once it's on.
- **Armani Luminous Silk Concealer (around £36)**. Tremendous.

- **Dior Skin Forever Correct (around £31)**. This is a beautiful concealer, with a very skin-like texture, that also works well under the eyes. Doesn't budge for hours and hours. Really creamy and comfortable. You only need a very little. Very good shade range for brown skins; merely okay for Black.
- **Fenty Beauty Pro Filt'r Instant Retouch Concealer (around £21)**. Huge shade range – we have Fenty Beauty, the singer Rihanna's makeup line, to thank for creating a completely inclusive beauty brand that was so wildly successful that it shamed other brands into following suit. This is creamy, long-lasting and buildable, and can be used on the eyes or face.

A special concealer note for people with brown skin

Not all Asian or even dark olive skins have yellow undertones. Sometimes it's more orange, which is to say peachier. If you have South Asian skin and have trouble finding a good match, particularly when it comes to concealer and even more particularly when it comes to under-eye concealer, try something that is more orange than yellow. It'll look weird in the container, but when it works on the skin, it's a revelation. This is, once again, to do with the colour wheel: if there's a lot of blue or grey in your under-eye circles, then the opposite colour on the wheel, meaning the colour that will counter the blue-grey, is orange. Yellow is good if the shadows are more purple, and something pinker will counter greenish tinges. Good orange concealers/correctors include **Charlotte Tilbury Magic Vanish in Tan, or Deep if you're very dark (around £26)** (both lurid in the pan, but trust the process); **Bobbi Brown Creamy Corrector in Dark Peach (around £25)**; and **MAC Studio Finish Skin Corrector in Pure Orange, only comes as a refill for the Studio Fix Conceal and Correct Pro palette in Dark (around £32)**, which is well worth buying; the shades are dark-skin specific and so deeply pigmented that they can hide tattoos.

A special note for everyone else

Don't go too light with under-eye concealer. Yes, it makes sense to brighten the area by going for a shade that is fractionally lighter than the rest of your face, but 'fractionally' means *fractionally*. And see page 247 for a more effective brightening method.

BB and CC creams

If concealer on its own isn't enough for you, try a BB or CC cream on top. BB stands for either beauty balm or blemish balm and CC for colour corrector. These were all the rage ten years or so ago, and although nobody much talks about them any more, they are brilliant if concealer or corrector alone isn't enough, if you don't have much to correct but fancy a little coverage anyway, or if foundation really isn't your thing. Crucially, they contain skincare, meaning they actively improve your skin as they sit there making it look nicer. They look gorgeously natural on, with your actual skin shining through, but improved. I love them. Note: I always apply these with my fingers – they wouldn't work with a brush, though it's never a bad idea to tap them in with a damp sponge after you've finished with your fingers. They are perfect for everyday.

THE EDIT: SIX GREAT BB AND CC CREAMS

- **Erborian BB Cream (around £41)**. It is very, very rare for me to try something on my face, look in the mirror and do a double-take. In the case of this cream, I did a double-take, then flipped the mirror over to the super-cruel, ultra-magnifying side. Still amazing! It comes in a tiny, unexciting, innocuous-looking little tube, but (a) oh, my God; (b) OH MY GOD; (c) unbelievably, it took thirty seconds for my skin to look better, as well as fresher and more youthful, than when I go through the whole lengthy serum, primer, foundation, concealer rigmarole. It is literally magic in a tube. What's more, being a BB cream, it's half makeup, half skincare, and serious Korean-French skincare at that. It's hardly makeup at all, really, and it's certainly not foundation, except for the astonishing fact that it gives you this absolutely incredible skin. The packaging says 'baby skin', which is creepy but not inaccurate.

A few things to know: the finish is matte, but peachy, natural matte, not dead-person matte. I far prefer this to the kind of base that gives you a wet-look face (see page 143), but if you don't, it's not for you. (Except it is! It's just so good! Just add highlighter if you want more glow.) Also, my skin is pretty decent on its own and I don't like a ton of coverage, which, as I've mentioned, I find very ageing. This cream also exists in a Super BB version, for people with acne-prone skin or those who want more coverage: since that's not me, I haven't tried it, though on the strength of the normal BB I'm inclined to recommend it anyway.

I initially thought the shade range was feeble, as is often the case with Japanese and Korean brands, though they are slowly getting better. There are only four. But as is the case with most BB creams, the shades seem to morph and adjust to match your skin tone – more weird magic. I am 'Doré', slightly too light in the tube, perfect on the skin. It's one of the best products I've ever used. The darkest shade, 'Caramel', would not in my view work on very dark skin, though the product is so good that it's worth a try.

They also do a **CC cream (around £41)**, which works as an ultra-light foundation and colour corrects, getting rid of redness and adding luminosity. The other jewel in the Erborian crown is the version of this that is for the body, called **CC Body (around £44)**, which is a body moisturizer that evens skin tone on the arms and legs, or wherever you want to put it. It is fantastic. If it's late spring and you want to get your legs out but feel they could look silkier and more even, this is for you. Great on upper arms too. Put it on, wait five minutes, then get dressed as normal. It doesn't transfer onto clothing. A great product.

- **IT Cosmetics Your Skin But Better CC Cream with SPF50 (around £37)**. Much fuller coverage than others of this type, but what coverage – natural, dewy, luminous, un-foundation-like, covers and blurs anything that stands in the way of perfection. Doesn't look heavy. Fourteen inclusive shades; also exists in oil-free and illuminating versions. Very good indeed.

- **IT Cosmetics CC+ Nude Glow Lightweight Foundation and Glow Serum with SPF40 (around £33)**. This contains 90 per cent skincare. The rest is a light, fluid cream, still providing quite a lot of coverage, but less than its sibling above. Glowy finish, as the name suggests.

- **L'Oréal Paris Age Perfector BB Cream (around £12)**. Has SPF50. Great texture, great dewy finish, lightweight and natural-looking while still blurring, hydrating, bargain price. Nothing to dislike here – except, why stick fragrance into it?

- **Dr Jart+ Premium BB Beauty Balm SPF 50 (around £35)**. Another one with a very high SPF, and lovely on the skin.
- **e.l.f. Camo CC cream (around £14)**. This one is full coverage, if that's more up your street, and is excellent. SPF 30, with hyaluronic acid, niacinamide, peptides and collagen, for well under twenty quid, plus it comes in a very wide range of shades that cater for all undertones. A really impressive product, though it's much more like a foundation than a CC cream to my mind.

Confusingly, some tinted moisturizers and skin tints are heavier than some of the BB creams above. But you don't need me to explain tinted moisturizers to you: they do what they say on the tin. I strongly believe that these and the BB creams are your most youthful options when it comes to skin makeup. There is no question of them ever appearing mask-like, or of settling in lines and creases. They let your skin look like a living, breathing thing, which is enormously flattering. If you've always worn foundation, do give them a twirl – they can look so much more modern and youthful. I know how tempting it is to keep thinking that all so-called imperfections must be concealed at all times – but as I said in the Introduction, that's societal conditioning: women's faces aren't supposed to look like dolls' or children's. Once again, I cannot emphasize enough how much less is more the older we get. Less makes you look younger. More is really ageing. I don't make the rules. (Don't despair if you love foundation – there are some brilliant ones around that won't make you look older at all. They're coming up after this.)

THE EDIT: SIX OF THE BEST TINTED MOISTURIZERS AND TINTS

- **Laura Mercier Tinted Moisturizer Natural Skin Perfector SPF30 (around £40).** This is the sibling of the concealer I recommended (see page 153), and has replaced its cult predecessor, which was amazing but came out in the late 1990s and hadn't had an upgrade. It now contains skincare and zero parabens. Very light and natural, dewy, radiant, perhaps too sheer for some. I think it's just beautiful on the skin. This is for you if you're broadly happy with your skin and are just after a little extra zhuzh. Also comes in an oil-free version. Inclusive shade range.
- **L'Oréal Paris True Match Nude Plumping Tinted Serum (around £15).** Contains hyaluronic acid for hydration and a polite level of glow. I would call this a light foundation rather than a tint – it evens out skin tone beautifully and looks very natural. Six shades to cover all skin colours.
- **Ilia Super Serum Skin Tint SPF40 Foundation (around £45).** A misnomer: this is not a foundation in any accepted sense of the word. It is a fantastic, very dewy, very sheer tint – one of the first to launch, in fact, well before other brands got in on the act (because, as I keep saying, the current trend is very much

for skin-looking skin rather than 'I like your
foundation' skin). Hence, not for you if you like
full, or indeed medium, coverage, though of
course (see page 151) a good concealer gets rid
of the need for heavy coverage, and this
product is also buildable up to a point. Makeup-
skincare hybrid, and contains squalane,
niacinamide, hyaluronic acid. There's zinc oxide
in the SPF, which means it might look a bit
white when you first apply it – don't panic, it
oxidizes in under a minute once it gets out of its
bottle and hits the air, and then the colour is the
colour you bought. Inclusive shade range.

- **Hourglass Illusion Hyaluronic Skin Tint
  (around £40).** This one offers much more
  coverage and is more like a light foundation
  than a skin tint. It also has a plumping and
  firming effect, thanks to being stuffed full of
  hyaluronic acid, and has pearlescent pigments to
  impart glow (the good candlelit kind). SPF15,
  which is pretty low – but this is really beautiful
  on the skin so I forgive it. Feels very luxe to use.
  Few options for very dark skin.
- **NARS Pure Radiant Tinted Moisturizer
  SPF30/PA+++ (around £37).** I absolutely
  love this and cannot see myself ever stopping
  using it. NARS describe it as 'everything, for
  everyone'. It has skincare ingredients, including
  the beloved vitamin C (which brightens skin

with every use); it makes skin beam with health; it gives a lovely glow; it feels light on the face; it's sheer but not so sheer that you don't notice it's on when you look in the mirror. Great range of shades. Close to perfection.

- **Typology Tinted Serum with Vitamin C, Squalane and Aloe Vera (around £30)**. The super-minimal option. This is lightly tinted skincare. Very French, doesn't look like makeup, *isn't* really makeup, but subtly enhances skin that you are already happy with while giving it plenty of hydration and other goodness. I adore this product and in fact this brand (see also their lovely **Tinted Lip Oil, around £19**, ideal for the lipstick-fearing) but I want to make clear that the effect is discreet. Inclusive shade range.
- **Jones Road What The Foundation (around £42)**. It's in this section because it isn't really a foundation in the classic sense. It's an extremely hydrating tinted balm that merely *looks* like foundation in the jar. If you have dry skin, long for something that makes it look nourished and luminous but still recognizably like your own skin, hate the idea of any but the very sheerest coverage and want pretty much the most natural, no-foundation coverage it's possible to get, chances are you'll love this. Be warned: some people hate it because they feel it doesn't provide enough, or even close to enough,

coverage. As I say, it's more a tinted skin balm. Super creamy and rich.

- **Chanel Les Beiges Water-Fresh Tint (around £52)**. This is a hybrid of concealer and foundation, in the form of little droplets of pigment suspended in liquid that meld together when you pump the bottle. Weightless; feels water-like and refreshing on the skin. More foundation-y than tint-y, but super-light. Lovely for summer.

PART 2

Makeup

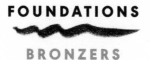

A lot has gone on in recent years, foundation-wise. A *lot*. I am always pointing this out to people who say they hate foundation, that they find it mask-like and obvious, and that they hate the feel of it on their skin. Mega-coverage, old-school foundations do still exist, but even they no longer feel heavy on the skin – and if, for some reason, that's the effect you're after, try **Maybelline SuperStay Full Coverage Powder Foundation Makeup (around £8)**, which is like kabuki and then some, but pleasant to wear. Generally, though, the predominant trend is for light, flexible formulas that are more and more like skin in a tube and less and less like the blanket-coverage, cakey-bakey horrors of the past.

Foundation should not be detectable to the naked eye, which means its texture should fit and meld with your skin's, not sit awkwardly on top. Most importantly of all, it should match your skin tone *exactly*. So many people still wear the wrong shade, which is a shame because a colour that's even fractionally off will spoil the whole effect. As I explained in the Introduction, I know how difficult it is to find the right shade. Not only did failing to do so make me feel like a freak, but it resulted in me wandering about in a kind of mad whiteface, or rather greyface, because the high-street foundations I bought gave me a terrible ashy cast. In retrospect I wonder why I was so determined to wear foundation in the first place – I had nice skin and not many spots – but I suppose it was to do with the teenage curse of wanting to fit in, to be and look like everybody else, including trotting down to Boots on a Saturday afternoon and buying horrible makeup that didn't suit me. Remembering this makes me feel really sad for my teenage self.

Every brand worth its salt now has comprehensive shade ranges, going from very pale to very dark – though, according to Black friends, often still not quite dark enough. And actually I don't find that the extended colours are always automatically all they're cracked up to be. I get sent whole ranges by brands and quite often pull out one or two shades thinking, 'Literally nobody is this colour.' I still often fall between two shades, too. But that's okay, I guess – it's certainly better than feeling excluded from a whole branch of cosmetics on grounds of ethnicity.

THE EDIT: THE BEST INCLUSIVE FOUNDATION RANGES

- All hail Rihanna, whom I have already mentioned and whose brand Fenty Beauty launched with forty shades of **Pro Filt'r Foundation (around £30)** – unheard of at the time. There are now fifty-nine shades, providing medium to full matte coverage, and fifty shades of the excellent concealer (see page 158). **Eaze Drop Blurring Skin Tint (around £27)**, also Fenty Beauty, is lighter and comes in twenty-five shades – said shades being quite elastic and forgiving, meaning there's likely to be one to match you even though the shade range looks smaller at first glance.

- **Charlotte Tilbury Airbrush Flawless Foundation (around £40)** has a matte finish, does not budge and comes in forty-four shades. My personal preference is for the lighter, glowier **Beautiful Skin Foundation (around £39)**, which I adore and which comes in thirty shades.

- **Pat McGrath Skin Fetish Sublime Perfection Foundation** is spendy **(around £61)**, but it's gorgeous – you can wear it as a skin tint, which looks beautiful, or build it up to a kind of low–medium coverage. Serum-like texture is lovely and light on the skin. Thirty-six shades.

- **NYX Can't Stop, Won't Stop Foundation (around £12)** is a brilliant budget option if you want full coverage. Forty-five shades.

- **Estée Lauder Double Wear Stay In Place Makeup SPF10 (around £38)** stays put for up to twenty-four hours and comes in fifty-four shades.

- **Lancôme Teint Idole, Huda Beauty, NARS and Hourglass** also make excellent foundations in wide ranges of shades.

THE EDIT: ELEVEN OF THE BEST FOUNDATIONS GENERALLY

All of these are reasonably inclusive, too, and they all have excellent staying power. Good foundations are usually expensive. You're paying for second-skin technology, which is always a plus but even more so on older skin. This is an area where I would actively encourage you to spend what you can afford – the results will be visible in the mirror. Skin is everything. There is nothing more ageing than bad foundation.

- **Charlotte Tilbury Beautiful Skin Foundation**, as above **(around £35)**. Great skin in a tube. That's all you need to know, except that it has tons of hyaluronic acid in it for plumpness and glow. Just enough coverage to make, yes, beautiful skin. Looks modern and fresh. I love it. Inclusive shade range.
- **NARS** are brilliant at foundations. My personal favourite, bearing in mind that I don't like too much coverage, is **Sheer Glow Foundation (around £38)**, which really is 'your skin, but better'. I have also had long and happy relationships over the years with **Soft Matte Foundation (around £31)**, which is as it

sounds, and more recently with **Light Reflecting Advanced Skincare Foundation (around £39)**, a skincare-makeup hybrid that is great on older skins and gives medium coverage. Inclusive shade range.

- **Hourglass** are also brilliant at foundation. If for some reason you need serious coverage that still looks like velvety skin, you can't do better than their **Vanish Seamless Finish Foundation Stick (around £50)**, which makes you look like an old-fashioned Hollywood star but miraculously doesn't feel, or look, cakey or heavy. If that's too much, I love their **Ambient Soft Glow Foundation (around £56)**, which contains 'blurring spheres'. This sounds like nonsense until you put it on, when you discover they're a real thing that visibly softens and blurs imperfections. Hourglass are very good at products that diffuse light flatteringly. See also their cult powders, page 214.
- **Make Up Forever HD Skin Undetectable Foundation (around £35)**. Makeup artists love this one, and I can see why: extremely natural medium coverage, sort of like a skin tint if it were a foundation. Says it's matte but isn't really – it has enough luminosity to be more of a satin finish. Inclusive shade range.
- **MAC Studio Radiance Face and Body Radiant Sheer Foundation (around £32)**.

This amazing foundation has been around for ever and there isn't a makeup artist in the land who doesn't have a bottle in their kit. You can make it look like the sheerest tint or build it up until you're ready for your close-up. It's as light as air and feels undetectable on the skin. You can use it anywhere – try it on your legs or arms if you're wearing something exposing and feel slightly mottled. Long-lasting, waterproof – it has everything. Outstanding shade range.

- **Chanel Les Beiges Healthy Glow Foundation (around £52)**. This one is just so lovely on the skin. Flattering satiny, glowing finish. Melds perfectly and looks ultra-natural. Not too much, not too little – just right. I can't think of anyone this wouldn't look beautiful on, at any age. See also their **Water-Fresh Tint** on page 171.

- **Il Makiage Woke Up Like This Flawless Base Foundation (around £40)**. This is a great medium-to-full-coverage foundation with a matte finish, but I'm also including it because it has an astonishingly accurate online colour-matching tool. I would always suggest trying foundation on in person (on your face! Not on the inside of your wrist or the back of your hand, which are completely different colours!) but in this case, you really can trust the online process.

- **Armani** is another brand that makes outstanding foundations, namely **Luminous Silk (around £40)**, and if you're after something very light, **Neo Nude Glow Foundation (around £34)**. **Luminous Silk** is a classic that is lightweight and silky, and contains technology that fills in small cracks. Absolutely beautiful on the skin.
- **Sculpted by Aimee Second Skin Foundation (around £25)**. Lightweight, lovely on the skin, looks very natural. Contains SPF 50 – bravo. Dewy finish.
- **L'Oréal Paris True Match Liquid Foundation (around £11)**. Contains hyaluronic acid for hydration. This feels and looks so much more expensive than it is. The colour range is particularly good for Black and brown skins. Very blendable; buildable medium coverage that will hide anything you want hidden without looking cakey.
- I almost didn't include **Bare Minerals Original SPF 15 Foundation (around £37)** because it's fallen so far out of fashion, but I have to mention it because, fashion or no fashion, it remains great, I still adore it and I still use and recommend it. This is a powder made up of ground minerals: the brand's tagline used to be 'makeup so pure you can sleep in it'. It looks like nothing in the little pot, but once applied to skin

(buffed in in circular motions with a very fat, dense brush; their own-brand one is good), it looks beautiful and utterly natural while perfectly concealing anything you want concealed. Note: you want the Original version of this, not the Matte, which in my view looks too flat on the skin. Wide shade range. It's worth looking up how to apply it on YouTube – it's a cinch, but you need to see how to do it before using it for the first time. After that you'll be able to put it on in the dark.

Applying foundation (and other cream cosmetics) to the skin

Having gone to the trouble of equipping yourself with the kind of excellent makeup that has the power to transform your complexion, it is important to apply it properly. Different tools give wildly different effects and levels of coverage. The following applies to all cream products, so concealer, blush, contour, cream bronzer, and so on, as well as foundation, though I am focusing on foundation in my explanations.

Fingers (clean) are great. You have them already, they warm the product up a little, which is never a bad idea, and they can get into every nook and cranny. You'll get a very natural, skin-like finish, so that's good. Identifying which bits of the face need more or less product is intuitive, and you can get it thoroughly into the skin, almost

massaging it in if necessary. Whether you're using fingers or something else, always start with the centre of
the face and work outwards – nobody needs a ton of
foundation or concealer on their temples – dotting on
less product than you think you need and really working
it in until you can't tell where it is any more. (It's easy to
add more, but a pain to remove cream products if you've
used too much.) When you've finished, wash your hands,
dry them well and press your outstretched fingers and
upper palms gently all over your face with a lightly roll-
ing motion, as if you were trying to get lint off a sweater
with a piece of Sellotape. This ensures that no rogue bits
of foundation remain unblended – the warmth of your
fingers will melt them in. The only thing that isn't ideal
about using your fingers is that a fair amount of product
stays on them, which can feel wasteful. But I am a great
believer in fingers as makeup tools (including on eyes).

Brushes. Applying foundation with a brush gives
fuller coverage, though this depends to a degree on both
the foundation and the brush. Natural bristles sound
nice, but they absorb product and are usually quite thick,
meaning they can leave weeny little brush-stripes (or the
odd bristle) behind. For this reason I prefer something
synthetic, and I prefer a round stippling-type brush to a
flat, more painter-like foundation brush. Stippling –
swirling and dotting the brush round and round, like
stencilling your sitting room in the 1980s – means you're
applying the product by making lots of little dots, which
eventually meld into a seamless (hopefully) whole. Flat

brushes can feel a bit like painting a wall with a nose sticking out of it, and I find it harder to get a pleasing result. I don't think I've used a proper foundation brush in years – they feel old-fashioned to me. Obviously if they work for you, then carry right on. I'm not the foundation-brush police. They're pretty much mandatory if you're using full-coverage stick foundation. Teeny-tiny brushes, the denser the better, are the best option with heavier cream concealers. Use a sponge, as below, afterwards if you can still see the brush lines.

Sponges. I mean Beauty Blenders, or any other egg-shaped makeup sponge. You hold these under the hot-water tap, squeezing a dozen or so times, until they've at least doubled in size, then squeeze them once more for luck and give them a final squeeze in a towel. They should be very slightly damp and fully plump from gorging on water, but not in any way wet. Then you dab them into a little bit of the product and bounce them lightly around your face like a Space Hopper. Boing, boing. Don't press or pat or drag. You just want the sponge to bounce lightly, which really presses the product into the skin (*you* don't have to press – it does all the work). Marvel at how a small dot of product goes such a long way! Gawp at the magical way it seems to bond seamlessly with your skin! Use the pointy end of the egg to get into the angles round your nose, eyes and chin, and the eggy end everywhere else.

These sponges spread the foundation (or whatever else) very, very thinly, in as many or as few layers as you fancy, and in doing so create an air-brushed effect. If you're wondering why someone's makeup looks so smooth and 'flawless' compared to yours, it's because they're using a Beauty Blender and you're not. They really make a huge difference. In case you're wondering, no, the sponge doesn't absorb the product, because it's completely stuffed with water and couldn't eat another thing, thank you, which is why it's so important to soak it properly. The only drawback of sponges is making yourself look *too* 'flawless', which can happen with heavier foundations or if you think, 'Wow, what a result, I think I'll go round again.' But I suspect I'm in a minority in considering that a problem. Other than that, I swear by them.

Note that you can also bounce a suitably dampened and squeezed egg sponge around your face if you've used your fingers or a brush and want everything to look a bit more seamlessly blended (but not as smooth as if you'd used only the egg in the first place). Eggs are also brilliant at getting rid of any accidental edges or lines by tamping them away – if you've been too heavy-handed with your blush, perhaps.

It's always important not to forget your neck when putting on foundation – it's naturally a slightly different colour – but it is particularly important when using an egg, because the contrast will be glaringly obvious otherwise.

I clean mine in a drop of blue Fairy Liquid, the anti-bacterial one, which gets it looking new again. (It seems to work efficiently only with blue Fairy, not green. Life is full of small mysteries.)

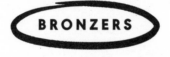

I'm putting bronzers here because I apply mine after foundation and before blush. I feel that doing it this way round frames the face, and then you can see where the blush, and whatever else you're using, needs to go. For me this works better than using bronzer last, when the rest of your face is already on. But each to their own! I don't apply mine in the shape of a '3', as is traditional, but rather horizontally, across my cheekbones and temples, which I find looks much more natural, then get on with the rest of my makeup. I revisit the bronzer situation when I'm done, at which point I often apply a tiny bit to my nose.

Bronzers are great but finding a really good one is harder than it should be. If you're using a powder, you want something very finely ground, texture-wise, so it diffuses rather than sits there looking obvious. And if in doubt, I would always go for something matte, but the *right* sort of matte – the wrong sort can look too flat. It needs to look lively in the pan when you open it – it needs to say 'summer' to you. If it says 'mud', it's not one you should buy. Don't go too dark. Bronzer is not fake tan. The idea is to look well, not to look like you nipped over to Barbados for the weekend.

THE EDIT: SIX EXCELLENT BRONZERS

- For me, the absolute acme of bronzers is **Chanel's Les Beiges Healthy Glow Bronzing Cream (around £37)** a cream-gel that is particularly easy to blend and comes in particularly beautiful shades – three of them, with the darkest not being dark enough for any but the lightest Black skins. They need a fourth, and maybe a fifth shade, to join the party. But I'm mentioning it because it's so lovely and so very easy to use – not at all a given when it comes to bronzers. Cream bronzers give a more diffuse effect than powder bronzers if you don't feel yourself to be skilled at blending, and I think they look more natural, too. This one makes it very simple to look as if you've spent the afternoon in the sun. You know that look, when it's been unexpectedly sunny and you've been out in it – your skin is glowing, not quite burned but prettily 'caught the sun', and there's a sort of halo of warmth coming off your face. Also, it gives a rich person's tan, which is a ridiculous thing to say, but I mean that this is a South of France tan, clear and golden, as opposed to anything muddy or even faintly grubby-looking, as some bronzers can be. It's not shimmery, quite, but neither is it entirely flat. It is perfection. If you prefer being bare-faced and don't hold with skin makeup, it's also absolutely lovely on a scrubbed face.

Apply with a blending brush, not too huge. (What is it with massive bronzer brushes? No wonder people struggle for the desired effect – you want a brush that is *dense* but not *giant*.) You're not swirling it on all over, as becomes unavoidable with too big a brush – you're placing it, carefully, anywhere the sun would hit your face, meaning the sides of your nose, your temples, the sides of your cheekbones, and a bit on the chin and collarbones if you're exposing them. My tip here is to buy the travel-sized version, which costs around £37 as opposed to around £46 for the full-sized one, which is massive and which you'd really have to be a bronzing fanatic to use up in a hurry.

- **Charlotte Tilbury Airbrush Bronzer (around £44) (and also huge).** There are several Tilbury bronzers – she's very good at them – including a cream one, but my favourite remains this OG iteration. Contains hyaluronic acid and very finely ground pigments to glide over skin gracefully without settling anywhere, meaning you get a veil or wash of colour rather than 'Here's my bronzer.' This makes it a cinch to use. Good shade range.
- **Jones Road The Bronzer (around £32).** A creamy-feeling powder that comes in gorgeous,

warm, realistic colours for a super-natural golden finish that it would be difficult to mess up. See also their **Gel Bronzer (also about £32)**, which is literally divine and imparts both colour and the prettiest, most wholesome glow. The definition of 'Wow, you look well.' Use the tiniest dot.

- **Guerlain Terracotta The Sun Kissed Healthy Glow Powder (around £46)**. I feel like Guerlain's Terracotta range invented bronzers, but I may be wrong. Either way, they do them wonderfully well. (The whole Terracotta range is worth exploring, if looking sun-kissed is your thing; they've recently added a very good foundation, too.) This one is a mosaic of four shades – corals, browns, peaches, tans – in a variety of textures. You swish a dense brush in the lot and away you go. They come in Light, Medium and Dark, and for Cool and Warm undertones.

- **Hourglass Ambient Lighting Bronzer (around £54 and about half that for the mini version, which to be honest is all you need)**. This is a mix of Hourglass's remarkable **Ambient Lighting Powder** (see page 214) with bronzing pigment. It looks a bit much in the pan, rather like a slice of marbled chocolate cake, except shinier. You will think, 'Hoo, no, that's way too dark.' But it isn't. It is just amazing on the skin – shimmery in the best possible way, like you were having dinner outside as golden hour was ending and the waiters were just coming out with tea-lights in jam jars. You can buy it solo – it lasts *for ever* – and it sometimes turns up in Hourglass's various limited-edition palettes, which are highly recommended because there are no duff components in them. Quite rare.

- **NARS Laguna Bronzing Powder (around £33).** These come in either matte or faintly sheeny versions, in a fantastic range of shades, including some for dark Black skin, and have a lovely texture, being ultra-fine milled. I like 'em any old time, but particularly when I already have a tan, which they do an exceptional job of enhancing. Having said that I always go for matte, I actually really like the sheeny ones.

Makeup

Blush is transformative. It imparts more life and vitality than any other makeup product. But I used to find putting it on well really, really difficult. I knew what I wanted it to look like – like I was blushing prettily and the blush was a natural, probable extension of my skin colour. Could I get it right? No, not for years. It always looked like I was wearing blush. Having finally cracked it, I'm sharing my findings. Good blush is about:

The shade. Since blushing is pink, I obstinately bought pink blushes for years. I love the idea of big rosy cheeks. But big rosy cheeks are not right for me, because there isn't any obvious pink in my skin. Pink is gorgeous, and such a youthening colour on very fair and very dark skin tones. On anyone with colouring from olive through to medium brown, though, peaches and corals might be more flattering and give a more natural effect. (Having said that, I sometimes like quite an unnatural effect, with the blush looking obvious and quite punchy, but only in the evening and only once in a blue moon. In which case I use a bright red blush, very carefully blended. A bright red blush can give you a kind of almost-sunburned look that is very pretty. You want, as below, something very finely milled.)

The texture. Creams sound like they'd be easier to blend, but this is not always true – some are so pigmented that they don't thin out sufficiently unless you use a comically tiny amount. I find powders are generally easier to blend, last longer and are better on oily skin. Some formulations are cream-to-powder. As with bronzer, you want your powder to be finely milled so that it diffuses rather than sits there in a big lump of colour that you have to blend for ages in an excessively skilful manner. There are also liquid blushes, in tubes, which tend to be slightly sheerer on the skin.

The pigment. Generally speaking, a lot of pigment, meaning a lot of dense colour per square millimetre, is a good thing, bringing vividness and intensity. But that isn't always true when it comes to blush, when you might want something quite subtle. You also have to decide whether you want shimmer or glow in your blush, or whether you want it to be matte. Matte is flatter and gives a more sculpted effect. Glow is livelier and fresher, but too much glow looks ridiculous on an adult woman of a certain age, at least to my eye. I've made you a list below that identifies blushes with just the right amount of gleam.

The application. This is obviously key. You need a really good brush for powder blushes, not too dense and not pointlessly huge – I like the Jones Road one – but I have found that my trusty egg-shaped sponge or, rather, a separate, dedicated egg-shaped sponge, makes applying cream or liquid blush an absolute cinch. Not to sound hysterical about it, but this discovery changed my blush life, turning a process that was pretty hit-and-miss into something guaranteed to work every time. I also like sheer-ish stick blushes that you can pat on with your fingers, especially for summer or holidays.

The location. This is the most important thing of all. When I was a teenager in the 1980s, blush went in a diagonal stripe under your cheekbone, blending optional. Quite the look – the blush was often a metallic pinky-purple horror from Miss Selfridge. Then in the 1990s we all learned about applying blush to the apple of the cheek, this being the fleshy part that springs up when you smile and that is roughly in line with the middle of your eye. Dramatic improvement! This looked fresh and pretty and far more natural than wandering about with purple stripes under your cheekbones. Everyone was very pleased with this discovery – so pleased that we all pretty much left it at that for the next few decades.

Here's the issue: things slide down as we get older. What looked perky and charming blush-wise when we were thirty-five now isn't flattering. The musculature of the face has changed. The apples have lowered, and possibly melded with the beginnings of jowliness or sag. We are placing our blush way too far down our faces, which has the effect of dragging everything down further. Blush that's too low on the cheeks also emphasizes nose-to-mouth lines or folds. The *numero uno* rule of makeup placement in older age is: EVERYTHING GOES HIGHER and ends on an uptick. (This is especially true of eye makeup, which we'll get to in a bit – you don't want to create any lines or shapes that droop even a tiny bit.) What I'm saying is, forget the apples. It's time to move on up.

I wish I could do you a drawing to explain this bit, but we're going to use our fingers instead. So: find your cheekbone, the bit at the front of your face rather than the hollow at the side. Press your finger into it and travel around it towards your ear: there's a hard protuberance under your eye, and if you follow it round back towards your hairline and go down a bit, there's a hollow. Can you feel it? Okay, so your blush goes at the end of the protuberance that more or less aligns with the outer corner of your eye, and diffuses mostly out and up towards the top of that hollow. It sits well above the (other) hollow of the cheekbone (the bit you suck in if you're pouting or making a beaky face to amuse children). It can travel a little bit towards the centre of your eye, but it mustn't reach it. And it certainly doesn't go under the middle of your eye in a great big cheery circle any more. Yes, it's much higher up and further to the side than you're probably used to. You're miles away from the apples. That's the point: it now lifts the face. You can even take it up and round a bit into the temple. Applying blush in this location makes a massive difference.

I don't know any really horrible blushes, to be honest with you – not in the way that I know some really horrible skincare or truly appalling foundations. Cheaper blushes tend to be less pigmented and thus to wear off quicker, but so what, really? Just put some more on again. This is an area on which there's no need to spend a fortune – though the expensive end of things includes some outstanding products.

THE EDIT: THIRTEEN BEST BLUSHES

- **Nars Blush (around £30 but also comes in minis)**. The formulations here are simply lovely. Some are shimmery, some are satin, some are matte. Yes, everyone talks about the shade called, sigh, Orgasm, though I find Orgasm's universality is exaggerated: it can look a bit orange on paler skins. I like Luster, a sheer golden apricot shade, and Torrid, a near-perfect coral. But you can't go wrong – the very wide range of shades are all beautiful and the website helpfully shows you what each one looks like on different skin tones.
- **Maybelline Cheek Heat Water Infused Hydrating Gel Blusher (around £7)**. This is great and a total bargain – a light, luminous gel-cream for a very natural flush.
- **Beauty Pie Supercheek Cream Blush (around £12 to Beauty Pie members)**. A nice fat little pot of pillowy, blendable rouge. The shade called Bare Blush is flattering on pretty much everyone.

- **Chanel Les Beiges Healthy Glow Sheer Colour Stick Blush (around £38)**. Lovely sheer-ish, easily blendable formula that is hard to mess up even when using fingers. Imparts instant wholesome healthfulness. Only three shades. I like the one confusingly called No. 21. Chanel also produces **Chanel Les Beiges Water-Fresh Blush**, which is beautiful (around £42).
- **MAC Blushes (from around £24)**. As with NARS, you can't go wrong here – MAC have a vast cornucopia of shades, finishes and textures, from the kapow! end of things to the sheer and subtle. Like a blush sweetshop. I really love **Sheertone Shimmer Blush** in Peachtwist, among many, many others.
- **Hourglass Ambient Lighting Blush (around £27 for the travel size, which is plenty)**. You may have noticed that I am extremely keen on Hourglass's Ambient line. It's based on their truly outstanding, luminous **Ambient Lighting Powder**, which you can read about on page 214, and which is fused here with a highly pigmented blush. The result is a lit-from-within, soft-focus effect that is exceptionally flattering. Three shades, all pretty universal. I like Luminous Flush. The amount of sheen is *perfect*.
- **e.l.f. Putty Blush (around £6)**. In case you're wondering: no, I haven't stuck this in here

because it's so cheap. It's here because it's so great. Cream-to-powder, plenty of pigment, lightweight enough to look soft on the skin, and comes, among other colours, in a great coral called Turks and Caicos.

- **RMS ReDimension Hydra Powder Blush (about £35)**. These feel like they melt into the skin and give such a great finish – the opposite of flat. They look almost alive on the face. The colours are uniformly great.

- **Dior Rosy Glow (around £34)**. Comes in six shades, including a scary-looking Barbie pink called Pink that is absolutely beautiful on fair skin – ignore how bubblegum-looking it appears in the compact. I love Coral and Rosewood for darker skins, and the bright red called Cherry is amazing on Black skin. Sheeny, glowy, packed with colour, but subtle in effect. Worth the spondulicks.

- **Armani Beauty Luminous Silk Blush (around £39)**. Really, really beautiful finish – it is impossible to tell where the blush ends and the skin begins, even if you're really bad at putting blush on. Ultra-finely milled, with an ultra-discreet glow. I use shade No. 50, a soft peachy-coral, and sometimes take it to the high points of the face too, like a bronzer. Also very much worth the spondulicks. It is dreamy: my favourite blush ever.

- **Sculpted By Aimee Cream Blush (around £16)**. Excellent brand all round, by the way, at an affordable price. This is a sheer cream formula that goes on dewy and soft and is buildable. Peach Pop is a very pretty semi-matte coral. It would be nice to have some darker/brighter shades.
- **Stila Convertible Colour Dual Lip and Cheek Cream (about £18)**. Blends like a dream and doesn't contain too much pigment, making it very easy to use. There's a lovely coral shade.
- **Jones Road Miracle Balm (around £36)**. This isn't, strictly speaking, a blush, though you can certainly use it as one. It is a new kind of multi-tasking product from the brain of Bobbi Brown the person (see page 205), who no longer has anything to do with Bobbi Brown the brand. It's kind of a skin enhancer, which sounds a bit vague but which means you can use it in lots of different ways. It's a tinted, hydrating, light-reflecting balm that is almost like solidified Vaseline in texture, or like lip balm. (You have to push your finger in to break the surface tension before you can use it. Quite satisfying.) The idea is that you apply it wherever you want a bit of colour or glow, or really a bit of life and vitality. It stops things looking flat or overly matte. The shade called Golden Hour is divine. I have

Tawny and sometimes use it as a blush and sometimes as a bronzer – basically, it's healthy-looking skin in a pot. This means that you can use it all over your face in tiny amounts and look like you're very well rested and just back from holiday – except that sounds like it makes you look tanned and is a summer product, which it isn't. It just makes you look ridiculously well. It's a balm, so it's moisturizing and hydrating and leaves behind the absolutely merest hint of sheen (like, tiny). You know how in movies people look attractive at the gym, all flushed with good health and vitality, rather than sweating like a horse and panting everywhere? It makes you look like that. It's one of those rare products that immediately become indispensable. I really rate it, especially for older skins that need a bit of oomph.

BOBBI BROWN

Everyone has a private pantheon of women they regularly honour in their head, and Bobbi Brown is in mine. A former makeup artist, she invented idiot-proof makeup. She also invented no-makeup makeup at a time when the fashion was for an almost kabuki-like mask. She made makeup for darker skins in the bad old days when no one else bothered, or when they paid lip service with one lone insultingly weird colour that literally didn't suit anyone. She understood the importance of skin's undertones at a time when one-size-fits-all concealers, foundations and powders were the norm. She used models of all ages and ethnicities decades before it was fashionable to do so. She made makeup for you and me – products for modern women who go out into the world and want to look like a natural, improved version of themselves, not as if they've painstakingly painted on their features for two hours. She made that effortless look achievable for everyone. She's done a huge amount in terms of making women feel confident about their looks. (One of her earlier pieces of advice was never to cover freckles, for example, which was radical at the time.) She is, in short, a genius.

Brown stepped away from her eponymous brand in 2016, went and did other things for a bit, then launched her new brand, Jones Road, in the US in 2020. It's now available here online. It's prime Bobbi – a small, hurrah, collection of life-improving, face-improving, easy-to-use basics that are, really, all you need. I strongly urge you to check out the whole lot. The colour palette is beautiful – delicious, hyper-flattering neutrals that it would be hard to go wrong with. Neutrals is a bit of a misnomer – they're neutrals that do stuff rather than sit there looking so subtle that you might as well not have bothered.

An important thing to remember here is that luminosity is not the same as glitter or sparkle. Luminizers make older skin look beautiful. They make it gleam with the suggestion of youth: younger skin shines in 3D; older skin is duller and looks flatter. If you've admired some-body's makeup, whether in daylight or in the evening, and not been quite able to put your finger on why it looked so charming and fresh, the chances are that it was because they had lit themselves really well using makeup. Light seeks light and bounces off it, so if some-one is glowing discreetly and catching the light in the most flattering way, it's likely down to clever use of lumi-nizing products. I know from my inbox that people find this whole luminizing-highlighting-glow-getting business a minefield but are keen to understand how to achieve the look, so let's delve into it. Many of the products I have already mentioned in Makeup contain built-in light particles, from foundations to bronzers. Now we're going to talk about stand-alone glow, the kind you put on with a brush, a sponge or with your fingers.

The basic principle is that a lot of makeup creates the illusion of depth, which involves creating shadows – think of contour, bronzer, even how you put on eyeshadow, with darker bits here and lighter bits there. Those shadows enable you effectively to reshape various bits of your face, by making some parts recede and others come to the fore. And that's all very good and useful, but shadows are, obviously, the opposite of light. Light is flattering, light is perky, light can highlight what you want to highlight, just as shadow can tamp down what you want to tamp down. So, when we use luminizing products we introduce extra light – to brighten things up, to emphasize certain areas, to make our skin, or cheekbones, or brow bones, or whatever, look luminous. I like it when you can't tell a luminizing product has even been applied. Done well, it can be hugely flattering. Done badly, it looks particularly awful, like there are random grease patches on your face for no reason, or just like you're insanely sweaty.*

What to use?

As ever, it breaks down into textures, finishes and colours.

Textures
Illuminating products come in lots of different formats. There are powders, creams, gels, oils, liquids, drops,

* If you are in fact insanely sweaty under your arms, Botox can really help.

glosses, wands, sticks, you name it, all of which contain light-reflecting particles and sometimes pigment too.

Cream formulas are obviously more moisturizing than powders, and arguably easier to apply, though there are exceptions. They are often, but not always, subtler, since the luminizing element is blended into a cream, which by definition diffuses it somewhat. They tend to have a dewier finish.

Powder formulas either come as a hard, baked offering in a compact, or loose. We won't go into loose here, because it has a tendency to go everywhere and life is short. But baked powders are great, provided they are applied to well-moisturized skin, which aside from anything else gives them something to stick to. If you are very dry, you're better off with a cream. Powders will unhelpfully emphasize dryness (this is true in general, not just of highlighters). Note that some – though not all – powders can emphasize textured skin. Once again, we're after something very finely milled.

Liquid formulas, like gels or oils, are also good on drier skins, and therefore liable to slide off oilier ones.

Finishes

I'm going to assume you don't want to look metallic or alien, so my recommendations are for lo-fi products that will make you glow prettily in natural light.

Colours

This is where it's easy to go wrong, because one size does not fit all. What is beautiful on one person's colouring will look silly or worse on someone whose colouring is different. Here are some rules:

1. If you're fair, go for pearl-like shades, so whites, silvers, palest pinks, or champagne.
2. If you're medium, go for peachy shades or those with *subtle* gold undertones.
3. If you're dark, you can go for goldier golds, all the way up to bronzes. If you're Black, play around and experiment – you can wear pretty much all of these.
4. If your skin has cool tones, don't try to warm it up with these products, it doesn't work – that's what bronzer is for. Stick to your lovely pearls and silvers, as above. Pinks add a degree of warmth, too.
5. If your skin has warm tones, don't use cool colours, like the pearls and silvers above. You can try rose gold if you want a bit of pink, but otherwise stick to warm shades like soft golds.

Where does it go?

On top of foundation, or whatever else you're wearing on your skin. Take a clean finger. Tap it gently into whatever product you're using. As with bronzer, we're aiming for the areas of the face that the sun would hit first. Tap a tiny bit of product on the tops of your cheekbones, the bridge of your nose (the bridge of the nose is really effective), and under your brow bone, unless your eyes are very hooded. Stand back and have a look. There should be a discreet healthful gleam. At this point you can also apply the smallest bit of highlight to the inner corners of your eyes, but I prefer to wait until my face is finished – sometimes I feel it needs it, sometimes I don't. You could also do your Cupid's bow if you want to emphasize your lips. *Minute* amount, if so: it looks lovely on the young but I wouldn't necessarily recommend it to middle-aged plus women, whose lips are not generally as plump as ripe cherries.

What you can also do now, though it is by no means always necessary, is get out a powder highlighter, tap a fluffy (but not huge) brush into it, and swoop it from your protruding cheekbone – the front-facing bit, not the hollow at the side – to just above your eyebrow. It is possible to do this with a cream product too, but I find powder sets better and lasts longer.

That's it! Nice, isn't it? We've just done a super-discreet version. If you like it, you can ramp it up as much as you want, especially in the evening. Next up, what to use.

THE EDIT: SIX OF THE BEST ILLUMINATORS

This could be a really long entry, but I'll keep it simple. I have tried dozens if not hundreds of these over the years, with wildly varying degrees of success. The list here consists only of absolute heroes.

- **RMS Beauty Luminizer (around £33)**. This cream formula is so, so good. Do you have fair skin? Get it in the shade Living Luminizer, a beautiful pearly white. Medium skin? Magic, a muted champagne colour, is ultra-flattering. I wear Peach when I have a tan. These are really subtle – you'll look like you have marvellous skin, rather than like you're wearing a cosmetic, and they're ridiculously easy to apply with a finger – just tap it on wherever you want it. Pleasingly all of these colours, pale-sounding as they are, work on Black skin. I'm mad about them.
- **Hourglass Ambient Lighting Palette (around £64)**, and worth every penny. I would not be without this, either. It's a trio of the best – much imitated, never bettered – illuminating powders, which you can use all over your face as a finishing powder (beautiful) or apply with a thin fluffy brush to wherever you'd like to look luminized. Unbelievably great. Comes in three colourways that should suit all skin tones.
- **Dior Forever Couture Luminizer (around £40)**. This is very iridescent, very long-lasting,

and comes in a really good range of six colours, pretty much guaranteeing an excellent match whatever look you're after.

- **MAC Strobe Cream (around £30)**. This highly iridescent moisturizing cream started the whole luminizing malarkey way back in the mists of time (2000). It is still great. Four shades. A little goes a long way. Sometimes I mix it with body lotion and wear a bit on the fronts of my shins.
- **Chanel Baume Essentiel Multi-Use Glow Stick (around £36)**. Not quite a highlighter, or maybe just a highlighter that's evolved. Imparts perfect radiant sheen that is almost otherworldly in its loveliness. Like, if you were in a forest and you suddenly came across a wood nymph, their skin would look like this. Sculpted or Golden are my recommended shades.
- **Glossier Haloscope (around £18)**. Contains powdered crystals, which give a subtle rather than a glittery shimmer. This is a big fat stick that glides on effortlessly and makes skin look gorgeous. I prefer it to several better-known big fat sticks, which can be A Bit Much.
- See also the **e.l.f. Halo Glow Liquid Filter** on page 142.

Contour

Please know that this is not something I am suggesting you use on a daily basis, or indeed at all. But it *is* quite interesting, contour. I became aware of it, like most people, when the Kardashians first hove into view: I became fascinated by, first, the Kim bottom, and, second, the insane amount of makeup they all wore, especially for people living in boiling-hot California. What really gripped me was that these industrial quantities of makeup sought to create a (completely unnatural) natural look: everything was skin-coloured, taupe, beige, brown, and they, or rather their makeup artists, effectively used these shades to significantly alter the old Kardashian features. They also used cosmetic surgery, as we all know, but let's ignore that. Contour seemed to have quasi-magical abilities too, and the fact of the matter is that sometimes, if you really need to look ultra-glam, it does have its uses.

The idea is always the same, whether you're talking about oil painting or makeup: dark colours make things recede; light colours bring things forward. Contouring is about creating flattering shadows. As an extreme example for illustration purposes only, if you have a double chin and paint it dark brown or black, then look at yourself dead on, it will appear to have receded. If you suck in your cheeks and paint the same dark brown or black into the hollow that appears, your cheekbones will look more sculpted and more prominent. Contouring is just a less extreme version of that. So, if you feel your nose is too wide, you can make it appear slimmer by drawing two lines down the sides and carefully blending them in; if you think your forehead is too big, you can shrink it by applying and blending contour up towards the hairline; if you want your eye socket to look more pronounced, you can add a little contour to the upper inner corner of the eye. The same principle applies to the jawline and cheeks.

If you're going to try contour (which is quite fun), there are just three things to remember: first, use a contouring cream that is a couple of shades darker than your skin and no more – some contouring products are ridiculously over-dark and make you look muddy. Second, blend very carefully with a dense but not too fat angled brush, or a sponge, always working upwards. Third: skinny contour sticks are much easier to use than great big fat ones, which are liable to go everywhere in an unhelpful way. Even so, contouring takes practice – don't suddenly decide to try it for the first time five minutes before you have to leave the house. But do give it a go if you're curious. It does work. Contour products are not interchangeable with bronzer, by the way: bronzer brings warmth; contour brings cool shadow. I don't use contour very often, but when I do it's **Victoria Beckham Beauty's Contour Stylus (around £32)**, on the basis that it's super-skinny and therefore much more wieldy; very good on the nose and eyes.

PART 2

Makeup

BASE COATS

CONCEALER

TINTED MOISTURIZERS AND SKIN TINTS

FOUNDATIONS

BRONZERS

BLUSH

HIGHLIGHTERS, LUMINIZERS AND
CONTOUR

BROWS

EYELASHES

EYELINERS

EYESHADOWS

LIPS

FAKE TAN

Hi, it's me, the brow evangelist. I can preach for England about brows, and bore for England too. They are incredibly important – they can completely and dramatically alter the look of your entire face. Every time I stop saying this and relax, under the assumption that everyone has finally got the message, up pops someone who *doesn't understand* and makes entirely avoidable, face-spoiling brow mistakes. And back I go to repeating myself, as I have done on this particular subject for at least twenty years.

If your face is a picture, brows are the frame. You wouldn't put an Old Master into a plastic frame from the pound shop. Frame your face properly, because brows *make* a face. A face with undefined brows just sort of peters out. The eyes float about unanchored and unframed. A lot of people think that mascara is the thing that makes the big difference, but it isn't. Brows make all the difference. You don't have to take my word for it: it's easily demonstrated. Fill one in and leave the other bare: there you go. Now quickly fill in the other, for Heaven's sake.

Young women by and large have excellent brows. Their mothers often don't. I hear regularly that they've given up because of some disastrous brow incident that took place when they were young, most frequently over-plucking. If that's you, I'm here to tell you: never mind. You can fix it. Right now, today. Whatever brow catas-trophe has befallen you in the past, it can be corrected using cosmetics.

Anastasia Soare* turned the world on to the import-ance of good brows back in the 1990s: her **Dipbrow Pomade (around £19)** is legendary (and recommended if you don't like pencils; use with a thin, precise, angled brush). **Brow Definer (around £24)** is fatter but impres-sively wieldy. Having been devoted to the pomade for years, I might now prefer the brand's **Brow Wiz (around £23)**, a very thin, very waxy, highly pigmented pencil that makes it possible to draw completely convincing individ-ual hairs. It stays put at least all day. The pomade is very good, and it covers a lot of eyebrow ground in a hurry, but the pencil allows for much greater precision because you're using a weeny little nib rather than a brush. This is the number one brow product in the US, and I'm not sur-prised. It comes in twelve shades – do give some thought as to which one you'll go for: too dark is never flattering, and that becomes truer the older you get. I would con-sider going one shade lighter than you think you need.

* Amazing woman. She came to the US from then-Communist Romania in the 1970s without a bean in her pocket and without speaking a word of English. In 2018, *Forbes* valued her brand Anastasia Beverly Hills at $3 billion; in 2022 they named Anastasia the thirty-eighth richest self-made woman in the US.

The best brow makeup

If you remember hard, scratchy brown pencils from years ago or, God forbid, if you're still using a little stub of one of those pencils, prepare to be amazed. Modern formulations are comfortable to use and very natural-looking. No one is going to look at you and think, 'Ah, I see she's put her brows on, then,' even when you have actually just put your brows on. Assuming you have some brows to work with, even really bad brows, you can have great ones. If you don't have any brows to work with, whether through alopecia or illness, or if you feel that your brows really are beyond salvation, or indeed if you can't be bothered with the daily faff of drawing them in convincingly, I very strongly recommend booking in with Suzanne Martin, @suzannemartinaesthetics, who currently works at the Lanesborough Club & Spa in London. She does semi-permanent makeup to an exceptional standard. People fly in from all over the world to see her. The brows she creates are described as 'couture brows', which seems about right.

I can't see your face, so I can't advise on the best eyebrow shape. What I will say generally is that a very arched brow is perhaps more ageing than a straighter one. As someone with naturally very arched brows it saddens me to say this, but filling in some of the arch does look more modern, partly because it looks less 'done'. (Bear this in mind if you have Botox that turns your arched eyebrows into Mr Spock's. A good practitioner should clock your arches and work accordingly, but these things aren't always 100 per cent predictable.) A very skinny brow is also ageing, which is a shame because so many people have gone through a phase of wild over-plucking at some point in their lives, only to find the hairs didn't ever grow back. You don't want great big caterpillar brows, obviously, but for most people something as natural-looking as possible is great – even if it's in fact completely artificial. This is the goodness and the joy of makeup.

If you have hooded eyes, brows can make an enormous difference by lifting the whole eye area. It is particularly important not to take the 'tail' of them out too far and not to have this tail pointing too much downwards, like a sad arrow, which compounds the impression of droopage. Straighten the tail out a bit and suddenly you have lift.

How to do your brows

First, the basics. Find a spoolie – if you use an eyebrow brush, there's probably one at one end of it: it looks like a little mascara brush. Brush your clean, unmade-up eyebrows into their natural shape. Now brush them back the other way. This reveals the gaps. Get a pencil, pomade, gel or whatever you prefer – recommendations follow – and carefully fill in those gaps in short little strokes, as if you were drawing in individual hairs, which in fact you are. Keep the pressure very light, as if you were sketching rather than doing the kind of furious scribbling that tears through the paper. Now brush your brows upwards. Any more gaps? Fill those in too. Then brush your filled-in brows down again, and into their normal, natural shape.

Stand back and take a good look. If you like your eyebrows and have them professionally shaped, or if they are naturally great, you can stop here. If you still don't like their shape or size or width, this is where you can cheat a better one. You do this in exactly the same way, by sketching in individual hairs above your natural browline. Don't make the inner corners of your eyebrows square, which looks very artificial and harsh: inner corners look best when they appear more natural, which means light wispy strokes to create light wispy hairs rather than a bolder, more felt-tip effect. And, as I've said, don't make the outer bits, the tail-y part, extend too far. Remember that any downward lines drag the eye down and make the area look sad and depressed, so don't draw the tail pointing too far downwards. Fill in part of the arch if it's very high, even if just as a one-off experiment – I think it makes a big difference. You should now have an excellent, natural-looking brow.

If you want significantly more eyebrow than you've got, or to significantly reshape the brow, start in a different way, by drawing a line in whatever shape you're after above your existing brow. Work from the centre outwards – the idea is to keep the ends as natural as possible, which doesn't happen if you start from either the tail or the bit closest to your nose. Fill in the gap between the new line and your existing hairs as above: tiny feathery strokes, using either a pencil or a pomade and a very thin, sharp-angled brush. Do the same below, again working from the centre to avoid a great unsubtle chunk of product at the nose end of things. If you want a very clean, graphic brow, you can then go in with concealer underneath the lines you have drawn to make things look super-crisp. (There are thousands of videos on YouTube showing you how to do all of this – sometimes visuals work better than words, and this is one of those times. Having said that, find someone whose eyebrows you like in the first place – some of the brows on offer are *a lot*.)

If lack of fullness is the issue

If you want fluffy brows and there just isn't enough material to work with, use a brow gel. They look like brow mascara and work by fattening your existing brow hairs with the aid of tiny little fibres, at the same time as adding colour and texture to any sparse bits. Then they dry, setting everything in place for the rest of the day. You are free to use these in conjunction with pencils if you want extra definition, or for shaping.

THE EDIT: FOUR GREAT VOLUMIZING BROW GELS

- **Benefit Gimme Brow+ Volumizing Eyebrow Gel (around £25)**. Does everything – fluffs, volumizes, tidies, colours. Very effective fattish brush. Water-resistant, long-lasting, six colours, including ginger and grey, though I would personally not match my brows to my hair if I were grey. I would always match them to the colour they used to be. Anyway: **Gimme Brow** is a classic for a reason.

- **Wonder Blading Dream Brow Gel Serum (around £15)**. This provides volume, texture, colour and a brow serum that boosts hair growth, plus it's water- and transfer-proof. Good dual-ended brush: one end spoolie, one end angled brush.
- **MAC Eyebrows Big Boost Fibre Gel (around £22)**. Excellent at creating fuller, fluffier brows in one sweep. Waterproof, sweatproof and comes in twelve colours. Quite a lot comes out on the brush – you might want to swipe it on a tissue before applying if you don't have a lot of brow to work with.
- **NYX Fill & Fluff Eyebrow Pomade Pencil (around £9)**. Waxy, highly pigmented, buildable, and with a clever mini paddle brush at one end to fluff everything up.

Eyebrow-growth serums

Do eyebrow-growth serums work? Yes, in the same way as lash serums (see page 237), albeit more slowly. But you have to be absolutely meticulous about applying them every night. Basically they interfere with the natural growth cycle, or rather the natural hair-falling-out cycle, which reverts to its normal pattern the moment you stop using the product. So it's quite a commitment, and quite an expense in the long term. For brows, I rate **RapidBrow (about £30: give it at least a couple of months)**, and **RevitaLash RevitaBrow (about £100, ditto)**. To be honest, impressed as I was when I tested eyelash-growth serums, human laziness means that it's ultimately a great deal easier and cheaper to just use a great mascara and a great brow product. It's not like there's any shortage of either.

THE EDIT: FOUR GREAT BROW PENCILS FOR SPARSENESS AND GAPS

- **Charlotte Tilbury Brow Fix (around £20)** and **Charlotte Tilbury Brow Lift (around £24)**. The easiest way of explaining these is that **Brow Lift** is like a creamy, waxy colouring-in pencil that will give you colour and definition, and **Brow Fix** is like a brow mascara that will add texture, then set your brows into shape. You don't need to use them both at once, but they make a pretty great duo.
- **Charlotte Tilbury Brow Cheat (around £24)**. A brilliant brow pencil for eyebrows that don't need anything dramatic doing to them. It fills

like a dream – it has an excellent precise nib, a lovely consistency, doesn't budge, and adds a perfect everyday degree of texture. See also her **Legendary Brows (around £24)**, which is like a less full-on brow mascara, i.e. a tinted brow gel, that, again, is perfect for everyday and for when you can't be bothered to fiddle about drawing on hairs. The teeny brush lets you be very precise.

- **Victoria Beckham Beauty BabyBlade Brow Pencil (around £30)**. Very well designed micro-fine nib for drawing the most convincing hairs, excellent creamy texture, perfect amount of pigment, long-lasting. I use this on myself most days.

PART 2
Makeup

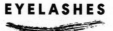

According to several surveys, most women's desert-island makeup product would be mascara. It's completely illogical – who would see it? – but it just shows how deeply we associate good eyelashes with feeling attractive. Heretically, I am not that fussed about mascara. I mean, I like it, and when I test mascaras I am frequently amazed at how good they've got in recent years. I used to be fussed – I was absolutely devoted to mascara, including electric blue and maroon, from the age of about fourteen, but since I moved to the country I no longer wear it every day. My own illogical (sunscreen and a decent shampoo would make more sense) desert-island makeup product would be brow pencil, which, as I've said, frames the face much better than mascara, which only frames the eyes. But I appreciate that this is probably a minority view.

Now, you don't need me to tell you how to put on mascara, but I'm just going to pass on this one good tip, which is particularly useful if the mascara you're using isn't brilliant. It is: put the brush at the base of your lashes as usual. Now don't move the wand up and down, but rather twirl it slowly on the spot. As you twirl, gently and slowly blink your lashes onto the wand. You might have to give it a couple of goes, because applying mascara in the normal way is second nature to most of us, but this twirling and blinking – don't rush it – results in much longer lashes. It takes a bit longer too, and you have to concentrate, or at least I do, but the results will make you go, 'Oh, my God, what?' One other tip: if you like the brush of a particular mascara but not so much the formula, rinse it clean and re-use it with the mascara you prefer.

Mascaras come in several different types. A quick reminder:

- Fibre mascara contains fibres, which are made of silk, rayon, nylon and sometimes cellulose. The fibres stick to your own lashes and make them very considerably longer and thicker. Fibre mascara is therefore great if your lashes are stumpy or sparse. They can flake a bit, and they can be annoying to take off if you wear contact lenses or have sensitive eyes. They're the best at giving a false-lash effect.

- Tubing mascara uses polymers that build a tiny little tube around each individual lash, which makes them longer, but not necessarily *much* fatter. Tubing mascaras are easy to remove with water alone. They are, like fibre mascaras, good at helping short or sparse lashes.

- Curling mascaras are designed for very straight lashes, though of course everyone else wants a curl too. These usually come with curved brushes and contain cellulose polymers to aid lifting.

- Volumizing mascaras prioritize girth over length, so the main aim is thick lashes. Their formulas are denser, waxier and may contain fatter pigments and silicone polymers.

Just to confuse matters, some mascaras do more than one thing.

THE EDIT: SIX OF THE BEST MASCARAS

Please see the application technique on page 233.

- **Dior Diorshow Mascara (around £33).** I don't like things being called 'iconic' when they absolutely aren't, but this really *is*. A brilliant false-lash-effect mascara that is like wearing lash extensions and gives sensational volume. Also available in a waterproof version. Dior mascaras are generally excellent, but this one is in a class of its own.
- **Maybelline The Falsies Instant Lash Lift (around £10).** The formula contains kera-fibres, made from keratin, as in human hair. Perhaps that's why the results are natural-looking, given the intense length *and* noticeable curling effect. (The brand says it's like a salon lash lift in a bottle.) Clever hourglass-shaped

brush with widely spaced bristles that give 'fluffy' lashes. If you have dead straight lashes, try **Maybelline Colossal Curl Bounce (around £12)**, which has 'memory curl technology' – no eyelash curler required. Good volume too.

- **Lancôme Lash Idole (around £25)**. A pretty perfect mascara. It lengthens beautifully, but not so much that you feel like you're wearing false lashes. It is brilliant at keeping lashes unclumped and separate. The curved brush delivers a nice amount of lift. The effect is wide-eyed and soft. The ideal everyday mascara. Lancôme make brilliant mascaras, so if that's not quite the look you're going for, try another – there isn't a bad one.

- **MAC Stack Mascara (around £26)**. This is particularly good if your lashes are small and stumpy. The clever brush catches every single lash, and you can even buy it in a Microbrush version for really titchy lashes, or for bottom ones. Volumizing and lengthening (it has fibres), plus impressively buildable – you can keep on layering it and it still won't clump or flake off. MAC also make a very good 'false lash' mascara called **Magic Extension (around £22)**, which comes in a really dark, intense black (not all blacks are the same) and which is for you if you want high drama. In a similar vein, **Urban Decay's Perversion Mascara (around £25)** is the business if you're after an 'onstage at the KitKat Club in Berlin in the early 1930s' vibe, in which case I, typing in my jogging bottoms *and* gardening apron, take my hat off to you.

- **Too Faced Better Than Sex Mascara (around £25)**. New mascaras come and go, but this one continues to have a fanatical following. I think it might be in the truly excellent brush, but the formula is no slouch either. It does everything – thickens, curls, lengthens like a dream.

- **Beauty Pie Über-Volume™ Fibre Lash-Building Primer + (£8 to Beauty Pie members)**. This is a mascara undercoat, designed to turbo-charge your trusty regular mascara. Contains fibres to lengthen and thicken, as well as 'lashwrap waxes' to coat each lash in volume and yogurtene for help with the curl. (I had to look 'yogurtene' up: it's 'milk fractions fermented with classic yogurt bacteria' and is good at conditioning hair. I want to write a short story about Yogurtene, raised off-grid in a yurt by gentle, loving parents who play the lute every night after supper. She goes on to great things.)

Lash serums

Lash serums are a solution that you paint on every night. They claim to grow your lashes to impressive lengths. I used to be highly sceptical about them. Years ago I tried a lash serum from the US that sort of worked, up to a point. But there has clearly been some sort of lash-serum revolution while I wasn't looking because I was too busy not believing in lash serums. Because I have found a lash-growth serum that absolutely 100 per cent works. Normally I would qualify that by saying 'absolutely works, at least on me', but I know at least a dozen people on whom it's worked too, and there are tens of thousands online. Of those dozen people, four had been urging me to try **UKLash Eyelash Serum (around £30 for a month's supply)** for months and months, and I hadn't, because I didn't believe it could possibly do what they claimed it did. But now I have, and I'm a total convert. There you are with your stumpy lashes, and there you are a month later with the kinds of lashes a good mascara can give you. We're talking length *and* fatness. It's nuts.

I'm amazed by this, and I don't really know what else to say, other than 'Get some.' Have a look at the before-and-after pics on the UKLash website. Having used the product, I really don't think they're retouched. From what I can fathom, and bearing in mind that the internet is incredibly unreliable when it comes to beauty products – sometimes the information is excellent, sometimes it's literally bananas, sometimes someone is being paid to say what the brand wants them to say and not making this clear – it works because of an active ingredient called prostaglandin, or a synthetic analogue that mimics it and appears on the ingredients list as isopropyl cloprostenate. It extends the natural growth phase of the eyelash follicle, which means the lash doesn't fall out but instead carries on growing. There's also biotin peptide, vitamin B5, another peptide that stimulates keratin, and so on. But the prostaglandin copycat seems to do the heavy lifting, and indeed appears in various other lash serums, though not in all – some rely solely on peptides. The peptide-y ones often say they will make your lashes 'healthier', as opposed to bonkers-ly long.

Now, the internet will tell you that some people find isopropyl cloprostenate irritating to the eyes, which I'm sure is true, but I have really sensitive eyes – like, sensitive to the point of hysterical: eyes that are constantly clutching their pearls and shrieking – and I am absolutely fine with it. The results are so extraordinary that, if I were you, I would buy a tube (it's around £30 for a month's supply) and try it. You'll know soon enough if it irritates you, and if it doesn't you'll be astonished by what happens next. You need to be patient – nothing happens for the first couple of weeks – or, at least, nothing happened for me. Week three is when it all kicks off, though of course your mileage may vary.

All you do is remove all eye makeup, let the area dry, then paint on a little line right at the base of your upper lashes, as though you were putting on liquid eyeliner, before you go to bed. Closing your eyes to sleep transfers enough product to the bottom lashes. One dip in the tube does both eyes, and they specifically say that's the perfect amount. Also you need to keep using this stuff, obviously, or the lashes will go back to their normal

'Think I'll fall out now' rhythm. But if you want longer, fatter lashes with minimal effort, you know what to do.

False Lashes

Bear with me. I know the idea of wearing false lashes as a matter of course sounds both hilarious and eccentric. But I was recently in London staying at a hotel ahead of a big function at an ungodly hour of the morning. The cab that was going to take me there was about four minutes away when I realized that the reason my eyes looked naked and mole-like, even though I was wearing a ton of eye makeup, was that I'd forgotten to bring my mascara with me. It was too early for the shops, and anyway I had no time, so I ran down to the hotel reception, explained the emergency and said that if a member of staff wanted to sell me their mascara, no matter how old, dried up or germy, I would buy it. Admittedly it was only about 8 a.m. and not everyone had started work, but out of all the young women who had, not one of them used mascara – they wore natural-looking false lashes all the way ('It's so much quicker and easier'). This claim will strike as borderline deranged anyone who's ever faffed about with lashes, tweezers and eyelash glue. Was I staying in a bordello?* Because 'easy' and 'quick' are not words one would ever associate with false lashes.

* When I still lived in London, for a while I used to go and have really good Thai massages at a Thai massage parlour in Marylebone. You can probably see where this is going faster than I did.

Believe it. False lashes are not what they used to be.

When the *Sunday Times* Style beauty editor told me fake lashes were having a moment, I said, 'Not in rural Suffolk among fiftysomething women they're not.' But no sooner had this conversation taken place than a giant box containing every single possible false lash available to personkind arrived on my doorstep, and I spent a very funny few days trying them all out. I made a visiting stepdaughter try them too. She is twenty, which is maybe more the demographic. Hilariously, we had supper in the kitchen, each sporting huge, very dark, very thick lashes. They looked like we'd stuck caterpillars on our eyelids for lols. I guess it's a question of context – it wouldn't have been especially funny in London but here, where the nearest pint of milk is a fifteen-minute drive away, it was completely absurd.

There was a time when I routinely wore false lashes on evenings out, but even then I always found them a faff. You'd get one on perfectly and think, 'Wow, so easy, I should just wear these all the time, they look amazing.' But then, without fail, the second one wouldn't play nicely. The glue would smear as you repositioned it, and then it would sit weirdly, or ping off at the inner corner, or start travelling as the evening went on. Then, years later, I became very keen on lash extensions for a while, an idea that now strikes me as so outlandish and decadent – lying there for ages with your eyes taped shut while some poor person painstakingly attaches individual lashes in the name of your vanity – that I can hardly believe it was something I did. Also, the process is intensely claustrophobic.

Anyway, it turns out normal false lashes – strip of lash, tube of glue – are still a faff for the above reason: sometimes you luck out and they both go on easily and look great, but it's random. There has been a massive improvement in the look and feel of them, though, and they are undeniably hugely flattering, especially if you're bad at eye makeup, because you don't need much else. The ones I liked best were by trusty Eyelure and are called **Lash Illusion Faux Mink Number 3** and **Luxe Velvet Noir Nightfall Matte Black Fibres (both around £10)**. Neither is subtle, nor subtle-adjacent, but the band on the Mink ones is incredibly thin so that if you do manage to get them on evenly, they look reasonably natural, where 'natural' means 'fell in a vat of lash-growth serum'. The fibre ones had a lighter texture. Obviously cut them to fit the length of your eyes, for God's sake, or they'll look mad. Equally obviously, they come in shorter lengths and less volume than the ones I tested. With one of these two, I can't remember which, I couldn't wear my sunglasses because the lashes pinged up against the lenses. I also got quite startled reactions shopping for groceries. But they do make your eyes look fantastic in the right context, and they are light and comfortable to wear.

The revelation was magnetic lashes. Lots of people do them but I liked **Lola's Lashes Hybrid Magnetic Lash Kit (from around £35)**. Again, they come in various degrees of length and density, from the relatively modest and plausible to the very much not. I loved these; they're such fun. You apply a liquid eyeliner first, which is magnetized, wait for it to be dry but still sticky, get a pair of tweezers and deposit the lashes (again, cut to size) onto the liner, to which they stick all on their own and where they stay politely all day and/or night. Obviously the success or otherwise of the enterprise depends on how well you can apply liquid liner, but since no one is going to see the competence or otherwise of your line because it's going to have lashes on top of it, even the cack-handed should be able to manage. Just make sure you stick to your natural eye shape. There's a good pen included in the kit that rubs out mistakes.

When you go to bed you just peel them off, ready to re-use (thirty-plus times, according to the brand). The only thing I would say is make sure you have some micellar water to hand. I didn't and couldn't get the liner off. I started freaking out about having magnetized eyes. Also, you're very aware of wearing these – you don't eventually forget they're there. I found them much heavier than the Eyelure, but this may just be me making psychosomatic associations between magnetic-ness and metal. They work really well, though, and they're as foolproof as a false eyelash gets. The website has useful information on what kind goes with which eye shape.

Recently I was telling a friend who was having chemotherapy and had lost all her hair that magnetic lashes might be the solution to the problem of her bald eyes, which she was finding challenging both aesthetically and because no lashes equals no useful dust filter. On top of everything else her eyes were constantly irritated and sore. So I dug out my massive box of falsies to pick some out for her, and in the process picked some more out for myself. They really are very easy to apply.

As I was saying earlier, I don't wear mascara every day. No, I haven't started wearing false lashes every day either, but do you know what? I now wear them all the time when I'm out socially. A couple of evenings later we were going out to dinner and I whacked some on – subtle ones, nothing too huge (Lowkey False Mink from Lola's Lashes, as above). I had no other eye makeup on. My eyes looked great. The density of the lashes acts as a sort of subtle eyeliner and, of course, the lashes themselves are quietly magnificent. They genuinely took under a minute to put on, which is actually less time than it takes me to put mascara on properly when I'm going out, what with waiting for each coat to dry. Do give them a go: they're just so easy.

PART 2
Makeup

BASE COATS

CONCEALER

TINTED MOISTURIZERS AND SKIN TINTS

FOUNDATIONS

BRONZERS

BLUSH

HIGHLIGHTERS, LUMINIZERS AND CONTOUR

BROWS

EYELASHES

EYELINERS

EYESHADOWS

LIPS

FAKE TAN

I love eye pencils. They are so easy to use, and make such a disproportionate impact. There's hardly any effect you can't create with them, from something very simple and clean to the full smouldering smoky eye, via everything in between.

Before we get started, though, I'd like to sing the praises of nude liner, which isn't usually white but skin-coloured now. Pale pencils have been used since the 1960s to create the illusion of bigger eyes, to remove redness and generally perk up tired eyes (I am repeating 'eyes' because I refuse to say 'peepers'), but they used to look very obvious – great thick lines of glaring white staring out at you, like Tipp-Ex. In their newer incarnation, they merely look pretty and still have a tremendous brightening effect. They are waterproof, since they sit in the waterline, this being the pink, fleshy part on the inside of your eye. A note: since nude pencils inside the waterline make eyes look bigger, it follows that dark pencils inside the waterline make them look smaller. Sometimes the smaller eyes are worth it – say, if you specifically want the full impact of a ton of kohl, top and bottom, or are going for a slept-in-my-makeup rock hen look. But generally, for every day, if you mind about eye size, then keeping the dark liner on the lashline rather than inside it is more flattering. Unless your eyes are huge, in which case there isn't an issue.

Knackered-looking eyes impact your whole look, so anything that wakes them up is a plus. As well as nude liners, I also really rate using eyedrops when you need to look particularly zingy – not all the time, because they get rid of redness by either constricting the blood vessels or limiting the supply of oxygen to the eye, which obviously isn't something you want as a permanent state of affairs. The best by miles are **Lumify Redness Reliever Eye Drops (from about £20 on eBay)**, which temporarily eradicate any redness, including veiny redness, as if by magic: they are incredible. They're easy to buy in the US but less so here, where you can find them online but where they are stupidly expensive. Still worth it for special occasions, though. Otherwise **Murine** and **Optrex**, readily available from chemists, do a decent job.

THE EDIT: FIVE OF THE BEST NUDE EYE PENCILS

- **Charlotte Tilbury Rock 'n' Kohl Eye Cheat (around £22).** A universal shade that is creamy, blendable and waterproof. Use inside the lower eyelid for brightening, or just below the lower lashline to make your eyes look bigger and more awake.

- **MAC Studio Chromagraphic Pencil in NC15/NW20 (around £17).** Also comes in two other fractionally darker shades. Creamy and soft, also waterproof.
- **Victoria Beckham Beauty Instant Brightening Waterline Pencil (around £24).** Whiter and brighter than the above, though not white-white. Very good.
- **Chantecaille Brightening Kajal in Nude (around £28).** This gives a slightly softer, smudgier effect and is a dream to use, as well it might be at this price.
- **Revolution Relove Kohl Eyeliner in Nude (around £2 from Superdrug).** I mean, it's two quid and it works. What else is there to say?

EYE MAKEUP AND THE OLDER PERSON

I have some observations to make about eye makeup and the older person. They are obviously generalizations, as for every woman who finds herself confused about what to use on her newly crinkly, increasingly hooded eyes, there will be another who doesn't feel her eyes are in need of special assistance. Admittedly I don't actually know anyone who thinks this, but they must exist. Anyway, a lot of nonsense is written about what older women 'should' and 'shouldn't' do when it comes to eye makeup, and it gets on my nerves. If there is one thing that older women know, it's that they are the boss of themselves, and have been around long enough not to take patronizing lessons about ageing from people young enough to be their children. So my first bit of advice is, do what you like. If it makes you happy and you like the way it looks, congratulations. You are winning. Don't let anyone tell you that you can't wear shimmer or glitter or bright colours, as if it were somehow unseemly and the only options now available to you are various shades of taupe. If you like taupe, and have always liked taupe, then sure, carry on with the taupe. (Taupe is good. I've nothing against it.) But if you used to favour something more adventurous, there is absolutely no need to effect a screeching U-turn, throw your beloved colours and textures away and shuffle sadly towards the world of beige. It is very bad for the health to stop feeling like yourself.

However, what you may find is that you'd like some guidance towards finding a happy medium, a way of still looking, and therefore feeling, like yourself, but one that is perhaps more considered and flattering than simply being on the same decades-old autopilot when it comes to reaching for the makeup bag. For instance, I used to like very vivid eyeliner, both liquid and pencil, in shades of violet or grass green as well as blackest black. I do still sometimes wear eyeliner like this, for old times' sake, but I have to be honest: it feels a bit much. I'm very conscious of my vivid violet line, and not in a triumphant 'Wow, my eyes look great' kind of way. More in a 'Hm, not sure' way, and occasionally even in an 'Oh, God, I think I might be wearing clown eyes' way. As I said in the Introduction, in older age there is quite a fine line between 'individualistic and confident' and 'wacky'. These things are subjective, but as I edge towards sixty, I do not want to look 'fun' or like a 'character'. The idea literally fills me with horror. I don't necessarily want to look ultra-elegant either, because I think it's terribly overrated (also boring, like being the human equivalent of pale grey paint), but given the choice between elegant and kooky funster, I'd pick the former. Happily, that doesn't have to be the choice.

To get back to my eyeliner: what I do now is a smudgy, nudey shadow base, some dark brown powder along the lashline, and a thin line of the green or violet blended out into the brown. The beloved colour is still there, hurrah, but in a more muted and frankly more flattering way, and now I *do* think, 'I like my eye makeup,' rather than fretting about its potential comedy aspect.

When it comes to eyeliner, and to making up an older face generally, I think it's a good rule of thumb to steer away from anything too graphic unless you're going for a very particular look for a very particular occasion (like a party with an eighties theme). Soft lines always look better than hard lines on older faces, and are way more flattering. A smudged pencil is sexier and more attractive than a harsh straight line drawn with an ultra pointy nib, and a smudgy eye is super-easy to achieve – just take a soft pencil, draw a thin line and, yep, smudge it (focusing the colour on the centre and outer end of your eye, to open it up and elongate it). I must also mention the lower lashline, because so many older women seem to think that if they line their upper lashes, they have to even things up down below. These things are completely subjective, but to me the eye looks bigger and softer when the bottom lashline is not drawn over with coloured eyeliner pencil. If you want more defin-ition down there, only line the outer corner. Doing it this way also allows you to use black, which is unbeatable in terms of drama and definition but can close up the eye and make it look severe if the line is carried all the way along the bottom lid.

Related: there isn't a single person whose eyes don't look fresher and more compelling if they dab on a tiny bit of luminizer (see page 209) or light eyeshadow with a bit of a gleam in it on the inner corner of their eyes, in that little gap between the inner corner and the start of the nose. I am also very much in favour of luminizer as eyeshadow, either all over or dabbed into the centre of the lid, over a neutral base colour.

THE EDIT: FOUR OF THE BEST PENCIL EYELINERS

I think it's worth spending what you can afford on really good eyeliners because they last a long time and there isn't another item of makeup that makes such a significant difference. I would go as far as saying that they are essential for all but the most makeup-hating. It is really easy for your eyes to sort of fade into your face as you age, which is such a waste of eyes and which can make your face look quite vague and washed out. Even a tiny, discreet bit of definition around the eyes makes a huge difference. Everybody has nice eyes for as long as they live: how often have you ever said, 'She has the most horrible eyes,' or 'His eyes are simply *disgusting*'? So it seems a shame not to dress them to their best advantage. However, you absolutely never want anything that drags the fragile skin around your eyes. These pencils are all super-soft and they all blend like a dream. Nothing is going to get snagged in any creases or make you feel like the whole thing is an uphill struggle with a depressingly poor payoff.

While we're on this topic: lining the bottom lid with eye pencil, as so many of us do on autopilot, is not always flattering because it can sometimes give the impression of dragging the eye down. It can also look harsh. Line the top lid with a pencil as usual, but for a softer option on the bottom lid, take a dark eyeshadow and a thin angled brush and line underneath the lower lash line, going about a third of the way across. You'll still get definition, but also a flattering softness.

- **Victoria Beckham Beauty Satin Kajal* Eyeliner (around £26).** The brand's bestsellers, and for a reason: these are great. They are super-soft and creamy, almost melty, and therefore a dream to smudge. They also come in a beautiful, highly pigmented range of really rich colours, both matte and shimmery. If eyeliner scares you, or if yours feels old-fashioned, these are your guys. Draw a line, which doesn't have to be precise or accomplished, along your upper lashline, as close to the lashes as possible, then flip the pencil and use the smudger end to smoosh it about, following the shape of the eye, keeping the line thinner at the ends and fatter in the middle. Work reasonably quickly, because it then sets. Easiest eye makeup ever. The shade Cocoa works on everyone; there are lots more, including two especially lovely and subtle greens and some divine metallics that catch the light but are in no way too much. And you don't have to smudge, obviously: you can also draw a neater line

---

* Kajal and kohl are not quite interchangeable, though kohls are often now called kajals. Traditionally kajals are softer.

and leave it at that. Even easier. I love these pencils.

- **Chantecaille Luster Glide Silk Infused Eyeliner (around £30)**. This is also a kajal, hence effortless gliding. It is silky soft. It comes in shades inspired by Fortuny silks. It's pretty fancy and extremely nice to use.
- **Charlotte Tilbury Pillow Talk Eyeliner (around £22)**. Also impressively glidy, though not quite as smudgy (the brand's **Rock 'n' Kohl** range is Smudge City, try the Smokey Grey or the Velvet Violet blended with shadow, as described on page 251). I really like this particular shade, which is a sort of aubergine brown. It doesn't sound especially appetizing written down but is a tremendously flattering alternative to black, which can look very harsh on older skin. Works on every skin tone. I also love **The Classic in Shimmering Brown (around £20)**, which is a perfect everyday daytime pencil.
- **Revlon So Fierce! Vinyl Eyeliner (around £8)**. This is *shiny*! Creates a glossy, long-lasting, waterproof line that looks like lacquer and gives an expensive, high-end finish. I know I was saying, 'Smudge everything,' only moments ago, but there are very occasional exceptions. I only know about this eyeliner because I saw a really quite elderly lady wearing it at a party and it looked so cool that I had to ask her what it was

('Excuse me, what's that on your eyes?' 'Sorry, darling, you'll have to speak up, I'm very deaf'). I think it's great for night. The really quite elderly lady was wearing a sober black dress and enormous pearls, FYI, which is why the vinyl liner (in cobalt!) looked so chic.

THE EDIT: FOUR OF THE BEST GEL LINERS

A gel liner typically delivers solid, deep colour in one fell stroke, sets and keeps it there all day. They can only smudge up to a point, they don't have the soft creaminess of the kajals above, and are also perfect for creating graphic lines, like liquid eyeliners except much easier to use. Some come in nice little pots to be used with a brush; some are gels in pencil form. The pots require fewer brush skills than you'd imagine, especially if you keep the line thin. What I like doing is drawing on a relatively neat line with a gel pencil, then going over that line with a softer kohl or kajal pencil, which I then smudge. Doing this means you get no hard lines or edges. You've got the gel liner in place and the softer pencil sticking to it, meaning you are guaranteed extremely long wear of the kind that wouldn't be possible with a soft pencil alone. Done top and bottom, it's a ridiculously easy way of creating a smoky eye.

- **MAC Colour Excess Gel Pencil Eyeliner (around £18.50).** Comes in lilac and cobalt blue (beautiful on Black skin), but also in ten other tamer, though not dull, shades. Punchier than the non-gel pencils above; perfect for drawing on a neat, clean line (and then smudging it a little, for preference). Absolutely doesn't move or travel to the inner corners to make those annoying little blobs.

- **Hourglass 1.5mm Mechanical Gel Eyeliner (around £19).** Super-thin, meaning it makes super-thin and precise lines. A super-thin line is the older eye's friend – you can get this right into your upper eyelashes, which makes them seem thicker and you won't necessarily even look like you're wearing it. Perfect for subtle definition. Great colours, including a deeply chic dark blue called Ocean Floor that is great on brown eyes.

- **Bobbi Brown Long Wear Eyeliner Gel (around £25).** If you like liners in pots, this one has in my view never been bettered. Highly pigmented, smooth and glidy, and not as hard to use as you'd imagine, unless you're trying to draw on huge feline 1950s flicks, which are often so difficult to match. Caviar Ink, a not-quite-black with a lot of brown in it, is very flattering. You can use this inside the eye as well as on the lid.

- **NARS High Pigment Longwear Eyeliner (around £22).** You can sharpen these, not always a given with gel pencils, which sometimes just twist up. Fantastic range of smoothly gliding, deeply pigmented colours in both matte and metallic shades. There's a dark navy called Park Avenue, which looks amazing on and always gets you a disproportionate number of compliments, given that it's just a navy blue pencil. Note: more people should wear navy blue on their eyes. It works with all eye colours and is more flattering than black and less expected (read slightly boring) than brown.

ONE LONE POWDER LINER

Of great specificity and genius, **Laura Mercier Tightline Cake Eyeliner (around £23.50)** is *the* most useful creation. It's been around for years and I hope they never stop making it. It's cake eyeliner, so a hard little circle of powder that you mix into a paste with water on the back of your hand with a flat eyeliner brush. Then you lift up your eyelid so you can see the pink underneath of your upper lash line and push the brush in between the lashes, starting from the middle and working your way to the edges. This is called tight-lining. It brilliantly defines the eyes and gives a different look from the same thing done with a pencil – it's both crisper and subtler. The line stays in place all day. Looks great on every eye, and is particularly useful on hooded eyes, when normal fat liner might be too much, or where there might not be room for it.

Fine on sensitive eyes and with contact lenses. A brilliant product.

Hooded or droopy eyes

Sometimes people are so cross with or demoralized by their recently arrived hooded or droopy eyes – or both! Wahoo! – that they think the doors of the eyeliner world have slammed shut in their face. Not so. Here is every-thing you need to know about how to make eyeliner work for you.

- Never put on eyeliner looking down into a mirror. Look straight ahead with your eye in its normal position, as if you were talking to someone. You want something that's visible when your eye is open and your eyelid is in its usual position. Otherwise what's the point?
- If your eyes are very hooded, the simplest thing is to apply liner to the upper waterline only, as described immediately above, using either the Laura Mercier product I just recommended (see page 258) or any other waterproof liner. This makes your eyes look bigger, your lashes fuller. Plus it doesn't take up any eyelid space.
- Nude liners (page 247) make your eyes look larger and more awake, hood or no hood.
- Another useful technique if the hood/droop/ crease doesn't extend the full length of your eye: line half of the eye, so starting in the middle

with a fine-ish line and thickening it slightly as you go along towards the outer end of your lid. The idea here is that if the inner corner already looks crowded due to overhang, cramming in some eyeliner there isn't going to make things look more airy. Just forget about it and start where there's more space.

- Also flattering on droopage: tight-line the inner upper lid as described, then take a dark eyeshadow and a very, very thin brush and line the base of your upper eyelashes with the shadow, keeping it as close to them as possible. Go *up* in minute increments, rather than straight along, and don't go down again. End on an uptick. Again, this also works if you ignore the inner corner and start in the middle.

- Remember: *always* end on a tiny uptick – any eye, of whatever age, looks depressed and sad if the line finishes pointing down, as it would if you lifted the pencil away when you reached the bottom outer corner of the lid. This is even truer if your eye naturally sags downwards: ending liner where the sag stops drags your eye (and face) down with it. Take the pencil back up a tiny little bit. You don't have to go as far as making a wing – stop at the point where you'd be starting it.

- If you're putting anything at all on any part of the hooded lid, always use primer. It will ensure that your painstaking work has something to stick to and that it doesn't transfer or migrate.

- You can make a proper dramatic wing if you'd like one, but in that case it's much easier to understand how by watching someone do it. The makeup artist Lisa Eldridge is always an excellent starting point for how-to videos, lisaeldridge.com.

- If you're nervous of using an eyeliner pencil or of trying out a new technique, use a powder shadow first to get the line and angle right, then draw over it in pencil. This is like tracing rather than sketching freehand and makes things much easier.

- Any mess or debris will close up the eye. Use a cotton bud to wipe away anything that isn't neat, even if you're going for a smudgy look. Smudgy doesn't mean you smear everything about and leave it – it still needs to end somewhere. The cleaner the finish, for hooded eyes, the better.

PART 2
Makeup

BASE COATS

CONCEALER

TINTED MOISTURIZERS AND SKIN TINTS

FOUNDATIONS

BRONZERS

BLUSH

HIGHLIGHTERS, LUMINIZERS AND
CONTOUR

BROWS

EYELASHES

EYELINERS

EYESHADOWS

LIPS

FAKE TAN

There is a school of thought that believes shimmer and sparkle don't belong on the lids of anyone over fifty. To reiterate what I said on page 249, this is rubbish. A high degree of shimmer doesn't *much* accentuate lines if you've blurred and filled them using a primer, but even if you haven't, anything that bounces light around a bit is such a plus that it's worth it. Matte is great, and it looks smart, but it's flat. Flatness does not look lively or animated – it just sits there, flatly. There can be something rather dusty-looking about a completely matte eye. I'm not telling you to cover your eyes with glitter, though please do if you'd like to, but rather to think about having a little bit of glimmer or shine somewhere on your eyelid to make the eye look more awake and more alive. Glimmer can make the skin of the eyelid look more elastic and juicier, rather than dry and immobile.

I personally favour matte shadow plus faintly sheeny eye pencil, but it works the other way around too, and I also really like a highly flattering simple wash of glimmery shadow in a neutral minky shade plus some mascara. The shadow and mascara draw attention to the eye, but not in a shouty way. The glimmer glimmers prettily, but it doesn't particularly call attention to itself.

The whole shadow effect is achieved in moments, with nothing more complicated than a finger. You might prefer to do this with matte shadow if your eyes are very crêpy. Maybe. I'd say 'sod it' and still go for sheen. A very effective way of illuminating the whole eye area without wondering about glimmer, shimmer, glitter and shine is to get a tiny brush (your finger is probably too big) and dot a tiny bit of product on the inner corner of the eye, as on page 252.

If you have hooded eyes and want to make optimal use of eyeshadow, do the same as you would with eyeliner, which is to say always put it on with your eyes looking straight ahead, in the position they would be in when you're standing talking to someone. At its most basic, all you need to do is take the eyeshadow higher than someone with a non-hooded eye, so that it shows when your eye is fully open. This method lifts the eye pretty effectively, given that all you're using is a bit of shadow and a brush:

1. Prime the whole lid.
2. Looking straight ahead and using a shadow that's a shade or two darker than your skin tone, and a small rounded brush, sketch a crease where you'd want one if your eyes weren't hooded. Go back and forth with the brush until you can clearly see this new crease.
3. Blend it very carefully by swishing your brush back and forth until there are no longer any

obvious harsh lines. You want the bulk of the colour to be on the outer two-thirds of the new crease. The inner third should be so well blended that it is barely there.

4. Go in again and, if you'd like, accentuate the outer third of the new crease with the same shadow.

5. Using an eye pencil, line very thinly under your upper lashes, pushing the well-sharpened nib of the pencil right up into the lashes. Remember! End on an uptick, not downwards. If it looks messy, smudge it carefully with a smudger or a small fat brush, still keeping the smudginess very close to the lashes.

6. If you fancy a bit of glimmer, put a tiny dot in the centre of the new crease area you've just created with shadow, level with the centre of your iris, and blend it well. Keep it in this central area.

7. With a fluffy brush, wash a pale highlighter colour under your brow bone. I would keep this matte, but only because I'm not personally a fan of shimmery highlighter on the brow bone – I think it looks dated. But you do you.

8. Add mascara.

That's the basic principle – you can ramp it up as desired and vary the colours and textures. For instance, you could use a much darker shadow for the fake crease, then go in with something slightly lighter beneath it. Some good eyeshadow duets that are useful for this technique and come in wearable nude and neutral combinations that are hard to mess up include **Trinny London Eye2Eye Tones (around £20)**; **NARS Duo Eyeshadows (around £26)**; and **Clinique All About Shadows™ Duos (around £24)**.

Here are the eyeshadows I like most for the older eye. The more expensive ones are worth it, in my view, but this is a category where you really don't need to pay top whack. There's a huge number of really good cheaper options. The main issue here is not having things sitting in creases. The following recommendations have all been tested specifically with this in mind, though I refer you back to Primers (pages 146–7) with regard to creases (as well as to dryness and discoloration): the whole point of primer is to create a smooth(er), more even area for eye makeup to sit on and adhere to.

THE EDIT: THIRTEEN OF THE BEST EYESHADOWS

- My favourite eyeshadow palette is **Victoria Beckham Beauty's Smoky Eye Brick** in the Signature colourway **(around £45)**. It's four complementary shades that are a cinch to use and with which you can create anything from a clean daytime look to a full-on night-time smoky eye. If stealth wealth or *Succession*-style

quiet luxury were a palette, it would be this one.
The formulations are fantastic too. I love big
palettes though I never finish eyeshadow
foursomes – I always find I like only some of
the colours – but I'm on my second of these.
Unheard of.

- **Jones Road The Best Eyeshadow (powder,
  around £24)**. Bobbi Brown's newish brand
  again (see page 206), and as we all know Brown
  literally invented understated, flattering makeup
  for women who want to look better without
  looking like they've tried. These shadows are
  lovely to use, long-lasting, and every single one
  of the fifteen colours is extremely flattering on
  an older face: you could close your eyes and pick
  one at random and you'd not go wrong.
- **Charlotte Tilbury Eyes To Mesmerize
  (around £26)**. These are little pots of
  shimmery cream shadow in pinky-minky-goldy-
  peachy tones. They are beautiful, impactful,
  long-lasting and ridiculously easy to use: stick
  your finger in the pot, apply to eyelid, done.
  What I like so much about them is that dunking
  your finger in the product and rubbing it on
  your lid – total time, twenty seconds – somehow
  looks like you've done something quite
  complicated and skilled. Older women often
  think they're not the demographic for Charlotte
  Tilbury, but that's incorrect. Beneath all the

high-octane darling-darling-mwah-mwah glamour
of the marketing are some really well-made, ultra-
wearable products that look great at any age.
This is one of them. See also the **Colour
Chameleon** fat pencils **(around £23)**, also
shimmery, which you can use as liners or
shadows as discreetly or fulsomely as you like
and which also give the impression that you've
done much more than you actually have, like
those really good recipes in which simple
ingredients miraculously turn into a dish that
has everybody exclaiming about the
unbelievable deliciousness.*

- **Kosas 10-Second Gel Watercolour
Eyeshadow (around £26)**. Same principle
from this clean beauty brand – idiot-proof
eyeshadow – but in this instance one that
gleams rather than shimmers. As the name
suggests, the finish is sheer and pared-back.
Swipe it on, wait ten seconds, then blend.

- **NARS Single Eyeshadows (around £17)**.
These come as powders and creams, as mattes,
satins and sparklier options. You can wet the
powder ones and use them as eyeliners if you
want to intensify the colour – this is true of all

* For me the queen of these sorts of recipes is Jane Lovett. If you don't
know her books already you will be very pleased that I told you about
them.

powder shadows and is useful because the finish is denser than if you'd used them dry but not as dense as if you'd used an eye pencil. These are excellent, heavily pigmented, long-lasting shadows in a ton of shades.

- **RMS Eye Polish (around £26)**. There are only two of these creamy shadows: one is a perfect minky taupe, the other a perfect minky brown. They have the merest, merest sheen on the eye, sort of as if you'd put lip balm on your lid. Really beautiful, universally flattering, requires zero skill to apply. RMS is one of my favourite makeup brands.

- **NYX Professional Ultimate Shadow Palettes (around £16)**. Specifically the one called Warm Neutrals, but only because they're the colours that I find most wearable. All of the NYX palettes are great – they have either sixteen shades **(around £16)** or a whopping forty **(around £28)** and contain mattes, satins, shimmers and metallics. I find the colour payoff excellent and the longevity more than adequate. These and the e.l.f. one below are really fun to play with if you haven't changed your eyeshadow in years and fancy trying something new.

- **e.l.f. The New Classics Eyeshadow palette (around £14)**. Eighteen modern classics in ultra-wearable shades and multiple finishes; also

Mad for Matte Eyeshadow Palette in Nude Mood **(around £10)**, which is simply brilliant and so chic; also **Bite Size Eyeshadow** in I Love You A Latte and Cream and Sugar **(around £4)**, which are mini palettes of four shades, matte and shimmering, in really well-thought-out colour combinations. You'd think the pigment situation wouldn't be up to much at these prices, but you'd be wrong. The shadows are also super-blendable. See also **No Budge Eyeshadow Sticks (around £6)**, which come in satin and matte finishes, and **No Budge Cream Eyeshadow** pots **(around £5)**, which also work as eyeliners when used with a brush *and* already contain primer. I love e.l.f.

- **Milani Gilded Nudes Palette 120 (around £29)**. Fifteen lovely shades in various finishes. Super-blendable, highly pigmented: you can't go wrong.

- **Revlon ColorStay Cream Eye Shadow (around £7.99)**. This stuff *does not budge*. They say it doesn't move for twenty-four hours – I've never tested that particular claim but they stay on perfectly from morning until bedtime. Mattes and shimmers in nudey colours that look and feel very luxe. Creamy and blendable, waterproof.

- **Maybelline Colour Tattoo 24 Hr Cream Eyeshadow (around £4)**. These are all

shimmery and easy to apply. They also do
not budge.

- **Urban Decay Naked Palettes (around £40)**.
I *love* Urban Decay's Naked palettes and have
done for the ten years plus in which they've
existed. Twelve brilliantly compatible, brilliantly
blendable, brilliantly pigmented un-boring
neutrals in a variety of finishes and textures.
Stone cold classic, with good reason.

- **MAC Pro Longwear Paintpot Eyeshadow
(around £18)**. Creamy eyeshadow that can be
as translucent or intense as you like and that
blends like a dream. Waterproof, ultra-long-
lasting, no creasing or caking, and you cannot
go wrong with the super-flattering natural nudey
colours. I've yet to meet a makeup artist who
doesn't have the shade Groundwork in their kit.
These are hands-down my favourite single
eyeshadows.

PART 2
Makeup

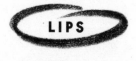

Lip shrinkage is real. Lips really bear the brunt of a lot of stuff. Loss of collagen makes them lose their stuffing, constant exposure to the weather knackers them – think of what the sun does to your face, and then think of what it must have been doing to your poor lips all this time. And that's to say nothing of central heating, cold weather, chapping and the like. Then there's the fact that we lick them all the time, not in a licky-licky come-hither way – or not *only* in a licky-licky* come-hither way – but as a matter of course, unthinkingly, whenever they feel dry, which is many, many times a day. I am also personally convinced that overuse of lip balm is a disaster for lips as it stops them thinking for themselves and makes them sit there helplessly, going, 'HELP! HELP! LUBRI-CATE ME!' rather than being self-reliant and sorting themselves out without making a giant drama (I also slightly think this about body lotion). I prefer using an occasional lip scrub – very easy to make at home by mixing a little bit of honey with some brown sugar, leav-ing on for about ten minutes and taking off with a warm

* 'Licky-licky' means crawling or fawning in Jamaican patois. It is such a good phrase.

flannel. If that sounds too complicated, even though it literally couldn't be simpler – and I am giving you quite a pointy look at this point – Lush will sell you nicely made variants on the same thing for about £7.

There's always filler. It can go very badly wrong if the practitioner puts in too much, not only because it looks stupid – it's the tweakment that most tugs at my heart-strings because if overdone it can look so *poignant*, so nakedly desperate – but also because the excess has a tendency to migrate. At the time of writing, many celebrities with various egregiously inflated body parts are having their filler removed; giant lips in particular seem to be on the wane.

That's not to say that lip filler – injections of hyaluronic acid – doesn't work, because when it's done well it absolutely does. Remember the tweakment mantra: only ever replace what used to be there; don't seek to create what never existed. If you've only ever had a normal-sized mouth, don't suddenly demand huge pillowy lips and be disappointed when they look grotesque. But there is such a thing as teeny-tiny lip filler that seeks only to replace lost volume and can work very well, provided there is still a decent amount of lip to work with. If you're planning to go down this route, it's extremely important to be completely confident that your top-notch, A1, not-cheap practitioner has a good eye. As ever, personal recommendations are by far the best way of finding such a person.

Most of us don't have lip filler or any intention of

having lip filler in the future. Still, thinning lips. What can we reasonably do? The first thing to bear in mind is that nobody has an obligation to have fat, plump lips where none are naturally available. If you consider your lips to be too thin or wrinkly for help, there is always the eminently sensible option of letting them be and shifting your focus elsewhere. Nobody zooms in on thinning and/or wrinkled lips if your skin looks great, or your eyes are amazing, or your nails are wearing a brilliant colour, or your earrings are charming, or, best of all, if you use your thin, wrinkly little mouth to say interesting things and make good jokes.

You can get lip balms with SPF, and they might be a good idea if, unlike me, you don't think that being addicted to lip balm creates more problems than it solves. I also have my doubts about how long they actually stay on for, what with eating, drinking, talking and licking. But I'd certainly wear one if I was skiing, or lived on a beach in the Bahamas. Otherwise, my solution is cheating. Over-line your lips, not in a grossly obvious 1990s way but using a pencil that is the exact same colour as whatever you're wearing on your mouth. Don't over-line wildly, obviously: we're talking a very tiny bit. But even a very tiny bit makes quite a big difference. Everyone I know who wears lipstick slightly over-lines their lips as a matter of course when they go out – why wouldn't one? It takes two seconds, no one can tell and it creates an impression of fullness, or at least of less thinness. You need a pencil with excellent staying power that's not going to bleed into any lines around your mouth, and you need to identify a lipstick shade (or shades) to match it (or them) with.

I can't be a great deal more specific than that since only you know what lipstick you like, except to recommend **Charlotte Tilbury's Lip Cheat pencils (around £20)**, all of which match her lipsticks. Everyone does lip-liners but I'm singling these out because Tilbury is most closely associated with a phenomenally successful lipstick shade called Pillow Talk, a pinky-browny nude that works extremely well when matched with Pillow Talk liner that has been drawn just beyond the natural edge of the lips: you really can't tell any cheating has gone on whatsoever. Pillow Talk is universally popular because it works on most people. It doesn't on me – it's too pale – but I'm not sure enough people know about its two siblings, Pillow Talk Medium and Pillow Talk Intense, which are great at 'nude' on darker, more pigmented lips. Nude is only nude if it's close to the colour of your actual lips: it doesn't have to say 'nude' in the colour name for it to be nude on you. Sometimes people forget this and, because there are a lot of bad nudes around, end up wearing a beige lip that effectively makes their mouths disappear, so that all you can really see is a slit and some teeth. There is no universe in which this is flattering.

To add insult to injury, a bad beige can make teeth look more yellow. Go for something with a bit of colour in it, and here I must make special mention of **MAC**

Crème In Your Coffee (around £20), a creamy, warm pink-brown that is not quite nude – better than nude, in my view – and that in my experience looks great on 99 per cent of people regardless of age or colouring. MAC are brilliant at nudes; see also Velvet Teddy and Kinda Sexy, among others. You can of course wear a bright-coloured lip at any age; the one thing I would say is that if your lips have become very thin, a really dark lip, like a red that is leaning into black, can look severe. Bright lips look particularly great – cool and modern – if you wear specs with heavy frames. This isn't a book about glasses, but I do think specs with heavy frames, ideally slightly oversized, are a great ally to all but the most fine-boned older faces. They're memorable, they're uncompromising, they provide a focal point, they frame the eyes, they look both classic and on-trend, and they have a kind of arty coolness about them that flatters the wearer. They say, 'Yeah, I wear glasses,' rather than 'Oops, where did I leave my little nana specs?'

Beware matte-matte lipstick: as I've observed else-where, matte can look flat and dead, and it can sit unflatteringly in lip lines. It also tends to be more drying, but if you love mattes, try **NARS Velvet Matte Lip Pencils (around £23)**, which are indeed beautifully vel-vety thanks to vitamin E and various emollients and won't dry your lips out. Generally, a bit of shine makes for subtler, juicier colour than anything dead flat. Soft shine adds the illusion of volume too. The trick is find-ing the right finish, whatever colour you like to wear, so your lips look hydrated and plump rather than startlingly shellacked.

For everyday, although I do still occasionally like a lined and very crisply defined red or pink lip, I prefer taking my favourite bright lipstick and smudging it on with my finger (see page 284). You still get the flattering, brightening punch of colour, but you lose the 'Hey, everyone, can you all please stare at my mouth' aspect that might be unwelcome if your mouth is wizened – not *literally* wizened, but you know what I mean. Not as pulpy as it was, let's say. With maybe some teeth issues and some smoker's lines to boot.* Smudged lipstick is also more relaxed, less try-hard, which is never a bad idea.

One last note on lipstick: if your hair colour has changed recently, revisit your lipstick. I'm thinking mostly of hair that is grey, white or any shade in between. I think it can look so beautiful and chic, but it can also wash you out a bit. For me, grey or white hair looks its freshest, most modern self when there is something quite vibrant going on elsewhere in the face. That could be a coloured eyeliner, a brighter blush or, easiest of all, a slightly amped-up lipstick. There's no need to go tomato-red (although, divine), but if you like a really nudey nude, for instance, maybe try something with a bit more pink in it.

---

* Isn't it *extraordinary* how much people used to smoke? On the bus! On the train! On *planes*, for Heaven's sake, and in hospitals! Whenever I remember it I am amazed by it.

THE EDIT: FIVE OF THE BEST LIPSTICKS FOR THE AGEING LIP

These are the best creamy, hydrating, comfortable lipsticks. The shades are up to you.

- **MAC Satin Lipsticks, MAC Cremesheen Lipsticks (both around £20) and Charlotte Tilbury**, as above; also take a look at **Tilbury's Hyaluronic Happikiss** range **(around £27)**, a lipstick-balm hybrid that is formulated with said hyaluronic acid for the purposes of intense hydration. Very pretty when it's on.
- **Elizabeth Arden Ceramide Ultra Lipstick (around £29)**. This is infused with the brand's Ceramide Triple Complex, which is designed to help with texture and hydration. Also contains something called Volulip™, described as an 'ultra-plumping agent'. Very comfortable on the mouth, perfect amount of sheen and, yes, slight improvement in plumpness.
- **Revlon Super-Lustrous Lipstick (around £7.50)**. A lot of colour for your buck, but feels very light and very hydrating on the lips.
- **Maybelline Color Sensational Lipstick (around £8)**. Comfortable and highly pigmented. I'm also including these because they have a shade range called Made For All that has been tested on fifty different skin tones and

that they claim will look beautiful whatever your skin colour – no guesswork required.

- **L'Oréal Plump and Shine Lipstick (around £9)**. Another lipstick-balm hybrid, this one providing mild plumping thanks to (pleasantly cool to apply) mint.

IN PRAISE OF SOLO RED LIPSTICK

as in, nothing else on the face

This has been my favourite makeup look for at least thirty years. It works on any age, but it does assume you're reasonably happy with your lips. You find the perfect red lipstick, which doesn't actually have to be a lipstick but can also be a balm, a lip oil, a balm-lippy hybrid – whatever you like. But it does have to be red. You put it on however you want to put it on, from very precisely, with a liner, to smudged on with a finger to blotted so it's more of a stain: you choose. And then you leave it at that. Now: this assumes a degree of confidence that not everyone is able to summon. In which case, you do the bare, bare minimum, the most no-makeup makeup imaginable: use concealer and maybe a BB cream, make sure your eyebrows are great, maybe put on one coat of mascara and the barest, most natural, best-blended dot of blush. Touch of luminizer on the eyelid. Then do the lip. Honestly, it looks so great.

There are so many self-tans on the market – an ever-expanding ocean of temporary skin dye, which is really what it is. The formulations get better all the time. Which is just as well. We're all aware enough of the damage to skin wrought by UVA and UVB rays to know that nobody should tan normally any more, as in on a beach towel, sighing with contentment. I'm afraid I don't always follow my own advice on this because I find it hard to completely shake off the idea that my brown skin, which has never knowingly burned, is more resistant to sun damage than if I were completely, rather than partially, white. That notion is complete rubbish, of course. I have the sun damage to prove it. Embrace the fake tan!

None of them will turn you orange now, but there are still gradations of colour, so it pays to do your research. (Ask around. I have really intense conversations about fake tan, usually with friends but occasionally with total strangers in the beauty aisles of supermarkets.)

In my view the wisest thing to do if you don't already have a fake tan that you absolutely love and swear by is to go for something gradual, so that you don't go to bed and wake up an improbable colour that you may or may not find pleasing – though gradual fake tans are also useful at prolonging the life of full-on fake tan. Now, obviously there are hundreds of gradual tans, and your mileage may vary depending on how light or dark you are in the first place. I like a bronzy result that, like my own skin, is quite olive, and that looks like I've spent a weekend at the beach in the UK, said weekend being pretty scorchio.

If you only want to even out your skin tone rather than go brown, see the excellent Erborian CC Body Cream on page 162.

THE EDIT: THE ONLY FOUR FAKE TANS I USE ON MY BODY

As ever, the finished result is closely related to the preparation, so make sure you exfoliate very thoroughly, whichever product you use. The quickest and easiest way to perfect pre-tan exfoliation is to use one of those inexpensive Korean skin mitts – search for 'Korean exfoliating mitt' online and dozens will come up. They're all much of a muchness, and revoltingly effective, in that you cannot believe the amount of dead skin they slough off using only water.

- I am very impressed by the whole **Bondi Sands** range, including its basic fake tan, which comes in various intensities, but I would specifically recommend **Everyday Gradual Tanning Milk (around £13)**. It would be very hard to go wrong with this one. It slides on really nicely, smells of coconuts and doesn't streak even if you're not super-forensic in your application – I just put it on like a moisturizer, which in fact is what it is: it leaves the skin nicely sheeny and hydrated and absorbs quickly (wait for it to be dry before you get dressed). It develops into a pretty, golden, won't-frighten-the-horses tan. There's a newer product called **Tinted Skin Perfector Gradual Tanning Lotion** – beige tube instead of blue pumpy bottle – (**around £14**), which starts working instantly and which I also really liked apart from the nauseating (to me) chocolate scent.

- If you'd rather cut straight to the chase and just go properly brown, rather than faffing about in the mimsy foothills of gradual tans, try **Bondi Sands Liquid Gold Self Tan Oil (around £16)**, which also exists as a foam but go for the oil. It's a dry oil, so it doesn't make you sticky, and it develops over two to three hours, with no need to rinse it off. It also smells of coconuts, and I find its oiliness gives it a slipperiness that makes it very easy to apply with a mitt. This is a good one to use if you're brown in the first place and find some fake tans don't show up as much as you want them to.

- **Tan Luxe (from £25)**. Tan Luxe make outstanding self-tan products. The

Illuminating Self Tan Drops (around, deep breath, £44), are amazing on the body. You mix them with your regular moisturizer, meaning you control the degree of tan that develops. I should say, given the price, that you don't use many drops. But their entire offering is good, from the mousse to the oil to the gradual tan. They also do an excellent instant tan, meaning it washes off, called **Instant Hero (around £24)**, which is very useful if the sun suddenly comes out and your legs still look wintry. Some instant tans are a strange colour. This one is perfect.

- **Saint Tropez (from £13.50)** make a ton of effective, well-loved self-tan products in a wide variety of formulations. My personal favourite is their **Self Tan Luxe Whipped Crème Mousse (around £26.50)**, which is super-hydrating and easy to use, touch-dry in moments and gives a lovely colour. Particularly good on uneven skin. Hard to mess up.

And the only two I use on my face:

- **Tan Luxe The Face Illuminating Self Tanning Drops (around £36)**. Lots of people do tanning drops but these are the best facial fake tan I've ever used. I am quite scared of fake tan on the face: there isn't much room for manoeuvre if you hate the outcome, and a lot of them sit in your pores, emphasizing them unhelpfully. This does not do that. As with the body version above, these are mixed with your favourite face cream or serum (I find a serum or face oil gives the best slip and a better result). Two drops make you look well, four drops make you look sun-kissed, and so on, up to twelve drops for the full 'just back from Mustique' effect. The colour is perfect: no one would ever think it was fake tan. Comes in Light/Medium and Medium/Dark. A brilliant product. **The Super Glow Self Tan Hyaluronic Serum (around £36)** is also recommended – same principle but with added glow.

- **Drunk Elephant D-Bronzi™ Anti Pollution Bronzing Drops With Peptides (around £31).** Not a fake tan as it washes off. But so useful and effective if you wake up wanting to look sun-kissed. Add a TINY pump (a little goes a long way) to your serum or moisturizer. Gives a very bronzed, very glowy effect; stuffed with skincare. I really love this one too. Very pale people might find it too much for the face. You can, of course, use it anywhere you like.

Speaking of fake tans: having chicken skin on your upper arms – its official name is keratosis pilaris – makes an even application challenging. The skin bumps are there because the tiny hair follicles are blocked. In this situation you want **Ameliorate Transforming Body Lotion (around £6)**, a genius product that deeply hydrates, gets rid of dead skin cells and unblocks hair follicles, thanks to the magic of AHAs. You need to use it twice a day for a month to see a proper difference. I don't love the smell, but you can't have everything. Also very good on ingrown hairs generally.

PART 3
The Extras Edit

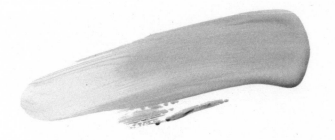

PART 3
The Extras Edit

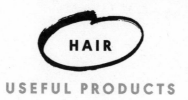

USEFUL PRODUCTS

Like eyes and necks, hair is one of the things that people ask me about the most. And so, while it's not technically skincare or makeup, it would be remiss of me not to include it in my *Beauty Edit*. Although this could be a whole other book, to be honest.

I really resent how much time I spend thinking about my hair. Having had a giant mane all my life and never given it a second thought, apart from to moan about how annoying it was to have too much hair, the post-menopausal thinning of my once-lavish thatch bothers me constantly. I should qualify that statement, before you start thinking that menopause makes you bald (it doesn't): I also blame stress and a predisposition to alopecia, which I once had in two 50p-sized spots, for quite a long time, in my twenties. But anyway: a friend took a picture from above the other day and I nearly died – I could see bits of scalp. My roots badly needed doing, which didn't help because white-grey hair next to the skin looks like baldness even when it isn't, but still, it wasn't at all nice.

My solution to this problem is extensions (for volume). They're not for everyone, but I swear by them. If you find the idea of permanent, bonded ones scary, go for tape extensions. Beyond that, **Toppik (around £20)** is a brilliant product if you have bits of scalp showing so, for example, if your parting is wider than you'd like – it's sort of like hair dust and sticks to whatever fluffy mini-hair is there, padding things out nicely. Don't go too dark or it looks weird. Go for very slightly lighter than your actual hair shade. For volume, though, extensions aside, there have traditionally been thin pickings. Texturizing sprays work up to a point, but aren't long-lasting. Dry shampoo, with or without colour in it, is a friend, because it adds texture and body, but it makes hair quite matte, and nobody wants to dry-shampoo every day. One of my friends deliberately bleaches her short hair to the point where it's so fried that it looks like there's a lot more of it than there actually is, but again, it's not a look that suits everyone, even if they don't mind the frying.

But salvation does exist, or as close to salvation as it's going to get. It's by **Living Proof** (whom I love), and it's called **Full Dry Volume & Texture Spray (around £30)**. You need this in your life if you have fine or thin or sparse hair, though obviously it also works if you don't and just want more of whatever kind of hair you have. You will have come across texturizing sprays before, but this is a whole new beast. Living Proof have a new patented molecule called 'volumizing & texturizing', and what's new about it is that, rather than bulk existing hair out by sticking to it, it creates space between hair fibres. This makes for big hair, but also, crucially, for volume that lasts. It's also very light, so that feeling of your hair flattening as the day goes on and it's dragged down by product doesn't happen. And it resists a certain amount of humidity too. It's got loads of grip. No residue, either.

You spray it on in sections at the roots, rub it in a bit with your fingers, as with dry shampoo, then muss up your hair as needed. (Shake the can between each spray or it doesn't work as well.) Seriously – three times as much hair. I couldn't quite believe it. It is still nowhere near as much hair as I used to have, but enough hair to have solved a situation that's been bothering me for ages. Utterly genius product.

With other hair products, I'll keep things reasonably succinct and just tell you what I especially rate, and why.

MY TEN FAVOURITE HAIR PRODUCTS

- **BEST HOME HAIR COLOUR**: Josh Wood Permanent Colour (around £14). I had occasion to try pretty much every home dye kit known to man and woman during the various lockdowns, and this is head and shoulders (har-har) above the rest. The colour is impeccable, the bits that come in the box – like proper gloves that don't tear or split – are great, the dye contains a conditioning complex that works as the colour takes, but no ammonia, and it leaves your hair feeling healthy and looking very shiny. Covers all grey. The website is full of useful advice and information.

- **BEST ROOT TOUCH UP**. Also **Josh Wood**, who does either a spray or one that comes with a blending brush. My favourite is **Brown (or Blonde) Root Smudge (around £15)**, which comes as a solid block in a little compact. I find applying this with the small brush provided gives the most natural finish: you can use it only where it's needed with greater precision. If you prefer a spray, the Josh Wood version is good too – I just find that all root sprays are too indiscriminate and always go on my parting, even when I've tried to avoid it, giving a Lego hair effect.

- **BEST AIR-DRY CREAMS**. Letting your hair dry naturally is always a good idea, if only to give it a rest from being tortured with heat. Air-dry creams kill frizz while adding texture, condition and shine. I like **Ouai's Air Dry Foam (around £26)** and **JVN Complete Air Dry Cream (around £23)**. JVN is Jonathan Van Ness from the TV show *Queer Eye* and, somewhat unexpectedly to me, his products are amazing. The **volumizing** range for fine hair is highly effective and the **Instant Recovery Serum (around £24)** is downright extraordinary: applied to the lengths of the hair, it turns straw into silk *and* it works on fine hair without weighing it down. If you're in the market for new hair care, this brand would be a good place to start.

- **BEST ALL PURPOSE CREAM**. To tame hair into shape, get rid of frizz, make dry hair look nourished, to add texture to flatness, add shine and generally zhuzh up your barnet on a daily basis, I love **Hershesons Almost Everything Cream (around £12)**. There are very few situations it's not useful in.

- **BEST 'WOAH!' HAIR CREAM**. **Color Wow One Minute Transformation Styling Crème (around £21.50)**. This stuff is like magic on dehydrated or frizzy hair. Works on dry hair only. Apply to achieve oomph any time; use to groom short hair so it looks salon-perfect; revive crappy-looking hair merely by putting a little of this on and working it through.

- **BEST BLOW-DRY TRANSFORMER**. **Color Wow Dream Coat Supernatural Spray (around £27)**. This is magic in a bottle. It basically laminates your hair, rendering it ultra-shiny and *waterproof*, meaning that humidity will not affect it in any shape or form, meaning frizz is dead and gone. Heat-activated. There is also a super-duper version called **Extra Strength Dream Coat (around £32)**. Whichever one you use, you need to be generous and really drench your hair in it. The results are amazing: you won't believe the shine.

- **BEST FIX FOR FINE, LIMP HAIR.** Equally magical, **Color Wow Raise the Root Spray (around £22)** gives limp hair astonishing bounce and body. Heat-activated.

- **BEST FOR COLOURED, MISTREATED HAIR**. The **Olaplex** range, which now includes mousses and serums, gives great results generally. If you buy one thing, make it **Number 3 Hair Perfector (around £28),** a pre-shampoo treatment that is a bond-builder – literally, it builds bonds where yours are broken, and in doing so eventually repairs your hair. You can actually see a difference after you've used it once.

- **A GOOD SERUM FOR THIN HAIR**. **The Inkey List's Peptide Volumizing Hair Treatment (around £14)** physically thickens each strand on application.

- **A LEAVE-IN HAIR MASK**. Arguably even better than Olaplex: a miracle potion called **K18 Leave-In Molecular Repair Hair Mask (around £18 from salons and online)**. This is a patented bioactive peptide treatment that heals and strengthens traumatized (because bleached, coloured, blasted with heat and heated styling tools) hair. Visibly reverses damage in four minutes. I wouldn't have believed any of this had I not experienced it for myself, but it's all true. Read the instructions, but in case you don't: you use this on towel-dried hair right after shampooing – DO NOT use conditioner.

- **BEST RANGE GENERALLY. Living Proof**, to reiterate, is an amazing hair brand, constantly researching and innovating. They are utter hair nerds, and as far as I'm aware there isn't a bad product in their entire range. Their own **Triple Bond Complex (around £42)**, which you leave in overnight, gives Olaplex a serious run for their money. Their dry shampoos are the best. Their normal shampoos are fantastic too.

- **MY FAVOURITE HAIRDRYER** is also by **Hershesons** and is called **The Great Hairdryer**. It is *tiny* and weighs next to nothing – about the same as an iPhone Max – meaning your arms don't get tired. But it's also powerful, contains technology to combat frizz, is super-quiet (for a hairdryer) and has a really long lead. It comes with a stand, a diffuser and two nozzles. It costs around £295. I was going to write that this is a lot, but in this age of £500 styling tools, it (almost) seems reasonable. It is just a brilliant hairdryer. If you don't have £295, I also very much rate **BaByliss's range of hair stylers**.

PART 3
The Extras Edit

HAIR

USEFUL PRODUCTS

- **Magnifying mirrors** reveal horrendous truths, but I think they become invaluable once you get to a certain age. If you've reached the fun stage when random hairs appear on your face overnight, you need one. The amazing thing about these hairs is that they are born adult, already measuring at least half an inch. (Despite their sometimes shocking coarseness. What's that about? Why is there basically a chest hair belonging to a very hirsute *man*, maybe in really small swimming trunks, maybe with hair also on his back, growing out of your face?) Anyway: they need to come out, obviously, but they are not always visible to the naked eye. You tend to notice them halfway through a dinner date, or just after a meeting. So the cruel, cruel mirrors are a must. There are loads of affordable magnifying mirrors for sale on Amazon and if your main purpose is hair removal, these are perfect. I would also get a small handbag version to carry about at all times. The crème de la crème of magnifying mirrors is the one by **simplehuman**, which has sensors and lights up the moment you peer into it. I wouldn't get this (or ask for it for Christmas) if my primary concern was the monitoring of rogue hairs, but it is very useful for putting on makeup, because the light it gives is the closest technology can get to natural daylight, meaning you don't put on your makeup in a badly lit bathroom only to go outside and discover it needs more work. This mirror, called **Round Sensor Mirror (around £200, less for smaller versions)** magnifies everything x 10. It's a lot. Maybe have a brandy before using magnifying mirrors for the first time. On the plus side, if your makeup looks good in one of these, it will look *incredible* in unmagnified real life.

- Related: good tweezers. I swear by **Tweezerman Classic Slant Tweezers (around £20)**. I've had mine for at least twenty years. They also do **a mini version (around £14)** that is good for handbags (alongside the pocket magnifying mirror) if constant hair vigilance is a concern. It certainly is for me. Get a brightly coloured one: they're easier to spot in the depths of a handbag and save rummaging about for ages.

- Also related: the best facial epilator is by Braun. It's called **Braun Face Spa** because it comes with a face-washing brush attachment **(RRP around £75 but it's often discounted** somewhere – **you should be able to pick one up for under £50)**. The face brush is fine but the epilator is the business if you can hack it. I have super-reactive skin that, tragically, can't tolerate any moustache-removing devices, waxings, threadings and suchlike – I go so red and blistery that by the time that's calmed down, the hair has grown back. I therefore use a kind of special lady face-shaver – which I swear doesn't result in beard-like growth appearing! – called **Finishing Touch Flawless Dry Cordless Facial Trimmer (around £20)**. I know, sexy name for sexy product. It's very good, though. It has a little light that illuminates the whole area where the hair is, so that you really can't miss.

- An excellent heavy-duty hand cream. Everything I've said about sun damage and faces applies to one's poor hands, which is why I always rub excess sunscreen onto them after I've done my face. As with the face, constant moisture is important too. I use three hand creams in rotation: **Avène Cicalfalte Restorative Hand Cream (around £11)** sits on my desk; **Lano Rose + Lanolin Hand Cream Intense (around £9, various flavours)** sits in my handbag; and **Nursem Caring Hand Cream (around £10)** sits by the front door. If I've been gardening without gloves, I sometimes rather melodramatically use **O'Keeffe's Working Hands Cream (around £8)**, which is for 'extremely dry, cracked hands', but better safe than sorry, I say. They also do a version for feet.

- Finally, a facial setting spray. These are like hairspray for makeup and ensure nothing even *thinks* of moving, sliding, melting or otherwise misbehaving. The best one by miles is **Charlotte Tilbury's Airbrush Flawless Setting Spray (around £28)**, which lasts for up to sixteen hours and is mildly blurring.

AND FINALLY: MY OWN SKINCARE AND MAKEUP ROUTINES

Don't feel you have to do *everything*. I've tried to be as comprehensive as I can be in these pages because I want to be helpful. But knowing all of this stuff doesn't mean I do it all myself. My own routine is very basic. In fact, here it is, in all its lo-tech glory.

In the morning, I wash my face with a warm flannel with nothing on it. I don't scrub like I'm a pan with stuck-on debris, but neither do I dab feebly. I put on sunscreen, whatever moisturizer I'm testing, and really massage it in, for ages, until it disappears, and then I leave it to sit and absorb while I brush my teeth and

shout at the radio. That's it. The whole 'routine' takes
about one minute. In the evening I remove eye makeup
with **Gatineau Floracil** (see page 20) or **Bioderma
Micellar Water (around £16)**. Then I clean my face
as if it were a military operation, often using **Emma
Lewisham Illuminating Oil Cleanser** (see page 18)
and my trusty flannel. I massage the cleansing oil in for
ages. I alternate between this and **Elemis Pro-Collagen
Cleansing Balm** (see page 18) , which I've used religiously for years. Once my face is completely dry, I use
Alpha H Liquid Gold three times a week (see page 31).
On the other days I use a serum, currently **Reome
Active Recovery Broth (around £75)**. Then I sit and
see what my skin feels like: I might seal in the serum with
a moisturizer, but in the summer I'd probably leave it at
that. In the winter, I also use an ultra-luxe facial oil, for
preference one by **De Mamiel** or **Alexandra Soveral**
(see pages 57 and 58). Either way, it also gets massaged
in carefully and for some time. Then I go to bed.

My daily makeup routine isn't much more complicated: on a normal day, working from home as I do,
I use sunscreen, concealer, maybe a BB cream, and
blush. I always do my brows. I will most typically
swoosh a dab of dull goldy-beige **Hourglass Ambient**
luminizing powder (see page 214) on my eyelids, even
though it's not technically an eyeshadow, tight-line
my upper lid with **Laura Mercier** powder liner (see
page 258) and add a non-dramatic mascara. If I'm going
out in the evening, I'll use primer and foundation, do

either more of an eye and a serious mascara (or false lashes, see page 240), or keep it as above and add a (normally soft, stain-like, but sometimes full-on) tomato-red lip. I always use my **RMS** luminizer (see page 214) on my cheekbones. I use it elsewhere too if I'm going out.

Afterword

I'm sure we've all looked at pictures of our younger selves and thought, 'It's downright tragic that I didn't realize how pretty I looked at the time.' From teenage-hood onwards, most of us spent so much of our life in a state of permanent low-level anxiety about being too fat, too thin, too tall, too short, too bosomy, too flat-chested, too straight-haired, too curly, too big-nosed, too short-legged, and so on and on and *on*, that we failed to delight in our own gloriousness. It is only ever later, in mid-life and beyond, that we can see ourselves as we really were – to look at our insecure fifteen-year-old self, the one who always compared herself to her friends and found herself wanting, and think, 'What was that all about? Look at me! I was lovely.'

So what I want to say is this: it will happen again. If you're fifty-five now, you'll feel the exact same way look-ing at pictures of your fifty-five-year-old self when you're seventy-five. You will think, 'I remember that time. I thought my eyes were too crêpy. How absolutely idiotic!' If you're sixty now, when you're eighty-two you'll look at images of your sexagenarian self and think, 'Ha, I remember myself then. I was obsessed with pores. I can't even *see* any pores. Cor, look at me in that dress.'

Society conspires to make women feel permanently

insecure about their looks and desirability at every stage of their lives. It's a load of old bollocks. Appreciate yourself *now*. Don't leave it until you're actually properly ancient. Your crêpy eyes aren't going to get any *less* crêpy with the passing years. Enjoy how you look *today*. Sure, you're not mad about your neck or your sun-damaged chest. Never mind. No one is. It's fine. It's not important. You're younger today than you're ever going to be again. Work with that. There are loads of little ways to feel good about how you look, and I hope this book has equipped you with a few of them. So there's stuff you don't like? So what? Celebrate the rest. Celebrate all the time! Because the alternative is always looking back with regret, and really, that is just pointlessly sad. Time is marching on. Choose joy!

Acknowledgements

Thank you to *Sunday Times Style* editors, past and present. Tiffanie Darke originally commissioned the column over breakfast after I'd droned on about how so much magazine beauty writing was just rehashed press releases and/or tied to various brands' advertising spend, and how as a cosmetics fan I found this irritating. Tiffanie's successors, Jackie Annesley, Lorraine Candy and Laura Atkinson, have all been wonderful to write for. Particular thanks to Sarah Jossel, *Style*'s Beauty Director, to Phoebe McDowell, acting Beauty Director, to chief sub Sophie Favell and to eagle-eyed Jane McDonald.

Thank you to Helen Garnons-Williams and the team at Fig Tree – Corinna Bolino, Kayla Fuller, Saffron Stocker, Ella Harold, Ellie Smith and Sara Granger. Thanks to Hazel Orme for the copy edit and to the beady pair of proofreaders, Sarah Coward and Annie Lee, and to Ben Murphy for the index.

And thank you, of course, to all the beauty PRs who keep me up to speed and awash in products.

Find me at indiaknight.substack.com

Index